Dreams Do Come True

Trudie Thompson & Lloyd Thompson

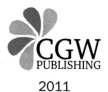

CGW
PUBLISHING

2011

Dreams Do Come True

The Amazing Story of One Family's Triumph Over IVF and Bankruptcy

Trudie and Lloyd Thompson

Original cover design by Jaja L. Thompson

Foreword by Professor Brian Lieberman

First Edition   September 2011

ISBN 978-1-9082930-8-4

Published by:

CGW Publishing
B 1502
PO Box 15113
Birmingham
B2 2NJ
United Kingdom

www.cgwpublishing.com

mail@cgwpublishing.com

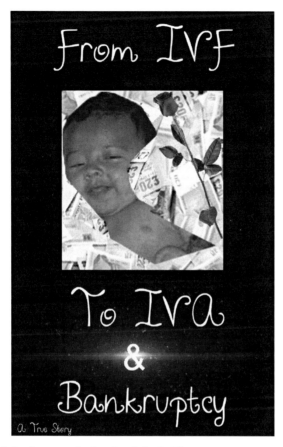

Original cover design by Jaja L. Thompson.

The Baby is me, on the original picture I was surrounded by teddy bears which I removed and replaced with £20 notes representing the money spent on IVF together with the money lost due to the bankruptcy but it also represents the return to financial stability.

The rose represents a bowl full of love, as that is all we need in life.

The Journey

Dedication

We dedicate this book to our beautiful son Jaja Lloyd Thompson who with the marvellous help of Professor Brian Lieberman and his medical team eventually entered this wonderful world on Sunday the 28th February 1999, the day our dreams came true and the day our lives began, he arrived at 13:14hrs weighing 6lb 6oz.

We would also like to dedicate it to every single child ever born; children grace this planet with pure wonderment, love, great hope, not to mention joy and laughter.

Our dream of having a baby was an all consuming passion that completely engulfed our world for twelve years. With hindsight, the pain and devastation we endured to reach our ultimate goal was worth every tear and was worth all the suffering. Perfection takes time and boy did we accomplish perfection when Jaja finally arrived. Every negative emotion melted away and we experienced what can only be described as ultimate love, the love every parent feels as their child enters this world and begins the journey.

Our dream today, our whole intention with the publication of this book is to create enough revenue to enable us to make continuous donations to St. Mary's Hospital in Manchester to support the birth of many more desperately wanted, precious babies.

Acknowledgements

We would like to thank so many people, but we obviously start with Jaja who continues to inspire us on a daily basis and who never even noticed how poor we became as the bankruptcy hit, for that Jaja we are both truly thankful. We thank you for creating the front cover of the book it really touched us that you wanted to be involved, again J thank you.

Sue, Michael, Jenny and Gerry, our totally wonderful selfless parents. We thank you for your continued support and your total belief in us. We thank you for your unconditional love and your help both financial and emotional, we feel very lucky to know you let alone be a part of your family, we are truly privileged and blessed. Thank you.

To Mike, my lovely Dad, a huge thank you for personally teaching us that you can overcome the most tragic of circumstances and stand tall and keep your dignity no matter the adversity. You are an inspiration to all who know you, (and thanks for theatre-land).

God Bless you Clinton, we love you dearly and we wish only pure health and peace for you in your later life.

My best friends, Christine and Gilly, thank you and bless you both for enduring my IVF years, always with patience and with kindness in abundance. Thank you for always making me laugh and for not being too proud to be acquainted with a bankrupt!

To David Graham Turner, you have been invaluable and you have never let us down. Thank you.

To Dr Sue Gelder, friend and Author of 'How I Cured my Tumor Naturally and How You May Help Cure Yours Too', thank you my friend for all your help and guidance, you truly are a pure genius.

Thanks to our siblings who are too numerous to mention but we thank you for just being you and for being there for us if ever we needed to call. Love you all.

Malcolm Wyatt, what a superstar! You were so kind and helpful, gently pointing us in the right direction and giving up so much of your time. Thank you for your patience Malc, and I promise never to darken your doorstep again with my begging bowl extended!

And finally, a huge THANK YOU to CGW Publishing, Christopher Greenaway, for having the faith and belief that we can actually pull this whole dream off. Thank you Christopher from the bottom of our hearts for believing in us and for giving so freely of yourself, you're a good man.

Dreams Do Come True

Foreword

The vicissitudes of life have touched Trudie and Lloyd. The ups and downs that they have experienced are typical of so many couples and they have overcome all these obstacles with fortitude and a smile.

I was delighted to play a small part in their lives. Children and, may I add, grandchildren bring great joy and happiness.

Raising children is a noble, time consuming and at times seemingly thankless task but there is no doubt that the effort is repaid many times over.

I have read their book and hope it will inspire many not only to go forth and multiply but also to keep trying in the face of adversity.

Brian Lieberman FRCOG

Emeritus Professor

Brian has been a consultant gynaecologist at St Mary's Hospital in Manchester since 1978. He is credited with the foundation of the first fully funded NHS IVF Unit in the UK in 1982.

The Sample!

Lloyd:

"OK Mr Thompson you need to provide a sample in this little pot"...

"Is this for real?" I was thinking as I took the clear plastic receptacle from her. She cut a rather motherly figure, plump, middle aged and bespectacled with a kind smiling face. She directed me towards the double doors at the end of the corridor and informed me I had been allocated room D.

Before pushing through the doors I had a furtive look back. It wasn't meant to be furtive but it must have looked furtive if anyone was watching because I was on my way to committing a most natural act in the strangest and most unnatural of circumstances that I could possibly imagine.

It was 9 o'clock in the morning and that was my saving grace. It meant that Trudie and I had got the first appointment of the day and no one else was around. Not even Trudie. She was in another part of the hospital being subjected to yet another series of tests. She was an old hand at this and was used to the various proddings of doctors and nurses and had even got used to the idea that on occasion the tests that were necessary were sometimes observed by teams of 'medical students'. She was desensitised to their presence as by now she was totally committed heart and soul to seeing this process through to a successful conclusion. We had no idea at that time that we were only at the early stages of a very long and winding road which was going to test us as individuals and as a couple. We had absolutely no idea.

"You will find some magazines in there to help you if you need them". She didn't just say that, did she? Why was there not a male nurse on duty? Surely that would work better in these situations? I swear she was smirking as she said it, or was my imagination getting the better of me?

I thought immediately of Trudie on a bed somewhere else in the hospital, 'legs akimbo' while doctors, nurses and an array of young wet-behind-the-ears medical students prodded, poked and rummaged around in their first medical tuition of the day! She always put a brave face on and visualised the end result and the joy and happiness we would feel when we emerged at the other side of this long dark tunnel. Sod it I thought, I can do this! If Trudie can go through all the necessary tests, treatments and operations, surely I can play my part. I was finally facing up to the fact that I was as equally involved in this process as she was.

One last look behind me, still the waiting room was empty and I pushed through the double doors and immediately across the narrow corridor, then I saw the room I had been allocated. I went in and closed the door behind me then locked it, then checked I'd locked it before checking it again. No I wasn't suffering from a bad case of OCD, I was making sure that no one was going to inadvertently stumble in here while I was doing my bit for medical science. How embarrassing would that have been?

It was obviously a hospital room but attempts had been made to make it look less clinical. There was a comfortable looking leather armchair, the lighting was softer than the normal bright fluorescents associated with hospitals and then there was the 'coffee table' with 'the magazines' to help me. I have to admit I needed help. I have never felt as unready in my life, and all sorts of peculiar distractions ran through my mind. Why was it so quiet? Who was in the room next door? Where was the hidden camera? Who was playing a drum at this time of the morning in a hospital? Then I realised the drumming was coming from inside me as my heart pinballed around my ribcage. For all I knew I could be playing the starring role in X-Rated Beadle's About! How long have I got? When will I be expected to appear back at reception with 'my sample?' How will I get said sample into this little pot? After all I'm a bloke who only has the use of one good arm.

Yet it's said that necessity is the mother of invention, which proved to be the case, as sometime later I emerged from the room proudly clutching the pot that contained my sample. I had done it! I felt like a seasoned IVFer!

I honestly don't know how long I had been in there but as I re-entered the waiting room my look of smug self-satisfaction dribbled away as I looked up into the sea of faces all looking accusingly in my direction. Had I come out with my flies undone? A quick glance South put my fears to rest on that one. No one uttered a word. There was total silence but all the faces were saying the same thing, 'We know what you've been doing'. Where had they all come from? There must have been half a dozen couples sat there looking at me. Where was Beadle?

Right I thought, brave it up and get out of here quick. After all it's not as easy to tell if a black person is blushing so, as long as my ears didn't spontaneously combust from the searing heat they were emitting, I should be OK.

Any hopes I had of just quickly leaving my sample and making good my escape in total anonymity were dashed as the nurse made me confirm my details to her and with great deliberation and volume repeating every syllable of my full name, date of birth and address as the silent hordes looked on! Why don't you just place an advert in the Manchester Evening News? Let's not settle for this tiny audience, tell the whole of the North West, why don't you, or should I just go round the room handing out business cards?

It dawned on me that the looks I was getting were from other couples in the same situation as us. In fact, as I studied the men without looking too obvious I could see fear in their eyes as they sat waiting their turn to go through the ordeal I had just survived. And that's just what it was, survival, making it through together. I vowed to myself there and then to give this thing my best shot and give Trudie the support she needed. If anyone could do this it was the two of us, and up until now she had been soldiering on with me playing just a minor role, a bit part. Now it was time for us to take centre stage together - Romeo and Juliet? Maybe not. Bonnie and Clyde? Probably. No, we would just be Trudie and Lloyd, parents to be.

Eventually I was released from my duties and set off to find Trudie. I had a bone to pick with her. "Oh you'll be all right, it'll be a breeze. You have nothing to worry about," she had said. Thing was, I had previously heard those exact same words, yet in much different circumstances. Trudie had a way of getting me to do the most unlikely things just by uttering those few words, and still does to this very day.

The Vision

Trudie:

"There! Look! Right there!" Lloyd was pointing at the monitor and practically jumping up and down. "Look!" he squealed as he frantically gesticulated in the direction of the computer screen.

At this stage I feel the need to explain that Lloyd isn't one for letting his emotions get the better of him. He isn't the type to wear his heart on his sleeve, and he most certainly does not breakdown at Bambi. But on this occasion he was wild and he looked completely out of control. And although Lloyd never cries, I could definitely see the well of tears. He was giddy with excitement. He never behaves this way, not unless Bolton Wanderers are involved. But that's another story.

I tried with all my might to focus on the screen the radiographer, Linda, had turned to enable a clearer view, which I hasten to add was a little more than a tad awkward from my horizontal position. It was totally useless. I just couldn't focus, and my own tears were making everything blurry, which exacerbated my frustrations. I was desperate to drink in the wee flicker Linda assured us was the heartbeat.

It was at this precise moment that I made my decision to jolly well stay horizontal for the next nine months, keeping my legs crossed and slightly raised at all times so as to ensure this little fella didn't fall out. This train of thought led me to wonder how on earth Lloyd was going to push this bed to the car park and how he was going to manhandle me into the car, maybe he could slide me through the rear door to enable me to retain my horizontal position, or maybe he could just tow me on the bed. Now there's a thought.

Just then something on the screen caught my attention. I saw the flicker. I actually saw that amazing tiny pulse, and it wasn't a figment of my imagination. I too wanted to jump for joy. I could not believe the euphoria that engulfed my whole being. My heart came alive for what felt like the very first time, it felt almost as if it had been swaddled in a fur lined hot water bottle. My pulse was racing and I was having difficulty breathing. Unbelievable. Surreal. It was only then that I truly believed that I, Trudie Anne Thompson, was actually pregnant. Finally after a lifetime of disappointment and longing, I was going to become a member of that oh-so-elusive club called 'motherhood'. Even though four weeks earlier the hospital had confirmed my pregnant status I just couldn't or wouldn't allow myself the pleasure of believing them. Plus I just didn't feel pregnant. There was no sickness, no tiredness. But now there was a flicker, and boy was I going to hold on to that image for the longest time.

Lloyd and Linda managed to eventually prize me off the bed, forcing me to my feet. I hated them for making me walk; it was much more comfortable lying cocooned on my safe bed. This was no time for the real world and having to do stuff, this was the time to lock myself away guaranteeing total immunity from the likes of chicken pox. As I shuffled, knock-kneed and pigeon-toed, down the corridor, I'd decided that this was my new adopted walk from now on, ensuring knees together at all times. And as soon as possible 'we' (baby and me) could sit and catch our breath. I didn't want to overdo things and take precious nutrients away from my unborn child. Poor Lloyd what was he in for?

As I shuffled, I directed Lloyd ensuring I didn't come into contact with another human being therefore avoiding all the potentially 'contaminated people'. I must stay sterile at all costs. Funny I should use that word – sterile - in this situation, but all I knew was that I had to get back to the safety of home and lock myself away, where I didn't need to let other people in and where I could just eat and grow. Grow! Now there's an understatement, but I'll mention my obesity at a later stage. Suffice to say Lloyd did once refer to me as 'his own beach ball with hands'. Cheek.

It was a beautiful summer's day in June 1998 and it would go down as the best day in history, or so I thought at that moment. But there was an even bigger event to come, one which would completely dwarf this moment. Only I just didn't know it yet.

I managed to make the front door of the hospital, Lloyd, bless him, had raced off for the car, leaving me unaided. I think he considered it the lesser of two evils, and I could see him legging it across the car park just as an elderly gentleman held the door open for me. I obviously looked too weak and far too frail and fragile to heave that heavy door. I must have looked as though someone had delivered me the last rights. He looked at me with his head slightly tilted to one side with a 'you poor thing' look in his eyes. So I just went with that. Well, I didn't want a conversation or anything and I wasn't sure what his ailments were. He was at hospital after all, even though it was a fertility hospital, which immediately begged the question, what would a geriatric type gent be doing here? Oh well, such was life, and so I shuffled past him. He must have been at least eighty-something, and there was me, a mere 38. He'd probably fought in the war. But hey, I'd gone through IVF.

With that, Lloyd pulled up in his car and clambered out, ran round to the passenger side and opened my door. I liked this pregnancy. It made all manner of people - even one's own hubby - open doors. I promptly shoe-horned myself into the seat with knees firmly together at all times, very lady-like, then as I sat there I thought, maybe I should ride in the back. You know, for safety reasons. Until Lloyd pointed out that he would look like my chauffeur, so I just stayed put.

Five minutes into the journey though I'm pretty sure Lloyd would have preferred me in the boot! We drove in silence from there, both of us lost in our own thoughts and memories of the events that had brought us to this stage in our lives.

The Meet

Trudie:

It was 1984 and boy we knew how to party, in fact we partied every night of the week I'm surprised anyone of us ever got to work, but we did, we just seemed to have the energy and we all held down very responsible jobs. In fact some of us had two or three jobs. I myself work at an insurance company during the day and behind a bar on the nights I wasn't out partying. No time nor inclination for resting, plenty of years that are set aside for resting, this was the time for burning the candle at both ends and in the middle too if you could.

There was a circuit of pubs and clubs we frequented so you were always bumping into the same people. On occasion though we'd vary our route and we'd change maybe the night or the venue. That way you wouldn't bump into the same people, sometimes for months. It was exhilarating it was fun and it was all about being young and carefree. Oh, and having cash to burn.

Obviously there were one or two fanciable folk on the circuit, and one such dude was Lloyd 'oh my God so gorgeous' Thompson. I must tell you that I truly had my beady eye on him, but then so did half the female population of Preston, Bolton, Chorley, Manchester. Shall I go on? No, you get the picture. Actually there was probably a large proportion of the male population that wouldn't have said 'no' to him either. He was what you would describe as pretty and handsome, sexy, trendy and heart-stoppingly gorgeous, very model-like in his appearance. And at that stage in my life I was very shallow and anything that looked that good was definitely gonna get my attention or anything else of mine he cared to take. He had perfect features, he was always smiling and laughing, he wore fabulous clothes and he hung out with the trendy people. More often than not he had an army of folk with him; never just one or two, he was without doubt 'Mr Popular'. Mind you, thanks to my friends I didn't hold out any hope of actually securing a date because, as they'd told me on more than one occasion, he was out of my league, way out of my league. Still I could fantasize. Where was the harm in that? And I could set my stall out too. Where was the harm in that? And none of my dear sweet friends need even know.

It was on one such evening that I bumped into Lloyd. I hadn't intended clubbing at all but I have very persuasive friends, or maybe you could say very manipulative friends. My friends desperately needed a lift to Cassenelli's, a club we frequented in Standish, so I drove them there and on arrival they forced me to go in for a drink. Well it would have seemed rude not to.

As we hung around the bar area waiting to be served, I noticed the delightful Mr Thompson and my stomach lurched, as it always did in his presence. Well, not even his presence, just the mention of his name could do the same. He looked over and nodded, I smiled back but then bad the dreaded thought that maybe the nod hadn't been directed at me. How stupid was I? Why would someone so delicious acknowledge the likes of moi? I mean how conceited am I? So I quickly looked away embarrassed and pretended to search for something in my bag, which was a big mistake as I was still wearing my 'ordinary' clothes with no handbag - no effort made there then, so why oh why did I assume that his nod had been for me. Sometimes my stupidity was in immense proportions and I knew that I had little hope of the floor opening up and eating me, so I decided to beat a hasty retreat and leave.

On my way out my closest friend dragged me into the rest room for a quick chat about some guy she'd been admiring. I listened intently, hoping I could appease her and make her feel better. She off-loaded her concerns and even though I tried to put my heart and soul into being a good friend, all I really wanted was to leave and get as far away as possible.

When we exited the loos the DJ was playing Roxanne's favourite tune, 'Somebody Else's Guy' by Jocelyn Brown. She grabbed me and shoved me towards the dance floor, pushing me through the throngs of sweaty people, and we squashed onto the edge of the rather packed floor, where I quickly conducted a scan of the surrounding area and relaxed as there was no sign of the lovely Lloyd. Partly for Roxanne's sake and partly because I too love that song, I threw myself into wild abandonment and I jigged and jogged with all of my might and sang at the top of my voice (yes we knew all the words – how sad) and to my surprise I was having the best time, so totally absorbed was I that I had almost forgotten the previous incident, until Roxy uttered those frightful words... "Don't look now but Lloyd Thompson is really checking you out"! At this point I completely froze. I was consumed by the dreaded thought that we'd come straight from the Ladies to the dance floor. Oh my God, I just knew that Lloyd was probably having a good laugh at the fact that I must be tucked into my knickers. Why else would he be checking me out?

The music seemed to go on forever and I was more than grateful when the following song wasn't quite so dancy. Roxanne was gesticulating that we should leave. What a relief!

Roxy was a real people person but also a totally free spirit. She was full of mischief and most definitely one of a kind. She was the type of friend that everyone dreamt of having and was extremely loyal, but she was always dreaming up ways to make life more interesting.

As we left the dance-floor Roxanne headed towards Lloyd's group. I could have died, what on earth was she doing? She knew the crush I had on him, for goodness sake. We'd discussed it on many a night over a glass or two of red wine. I didn't know what to do, so in true lapdog fashion I just followed her! By now she had already reached the group and started speaking to him, but due to the pounding of the music (or was that the pounding of my ribcage?) I was unable to hear what was being said. Just as quickly she then made to depart and headed to the bar for a top-up. She was so matter of fact; she'd just breezed in, had a quick word then breezed off. I couldn't wait to cross-examine her; I shrugged my shoulders in Lloyd's direction and smiled, relieved that maybe once I'd finished with Roxy I could just leave.

At that point, I decided to brave it as I was already stood there like a lemon, so I proffered the word 'Hi'. It wasn't like I'd never spoken to him before. Five years earlier I used to see him in Clouds nightclub in Preston and on occasion we would have a dance. Once he even held my hand as we left the dance-floor, a poignant moment in time that I would remember forever. But, although it was something I'll never forget, I shouldn't imagine it would have featured as a high spot in his life. So with this in mind I decided to bite the bullet and I asked where his 'long-term' girlfriend was. He replied that his relationship had ended. He then added, "It's good to see you Trudie, where's your boyfriend?"

Good lord, he remembered my name. My life was complete. Suddenly I was all aglow, feeling things I'd only ever read about in Mills and Boon or Danielle Steele novels! Those authors were bob on, they knew exactly what they were talking about, and it felt wonderful, be it a little scary.

"I'm not with him anymore". I was unbelievably grateful that I'd managed to speak, I was doing extremely well at exuding confidence, though I knew I wouldn't be able to sustain this performance and it crossed my mind that maybe he could see my palpitations.

Amazingly he proceeded to introduce me to his friends and he chatted away with great ease about who was who, and more importantly, who was with who. His brother Adam (who looked a lot like Lloyd) seemed more than an interesting character, full of fun, and the stunning, somewhat intimidating, women were all extremely lovely, very accommodating of me, nothing like you'd expect from women who looked like that, again very chatty. It seemed as though everyone was just happy to have made a new friend, I was honoured and my nervousness diminished ever so slightly.

At that point I explained my rather tatty attire and the fact that I'd only driven the girls for their night out, I wasn't staying. I babbled on for a minute, I suppose I was hoping that he'd be mortified by my suggested departure and beg me to stay. But of course he didn't, things like that didn't happen in the real world to ordinary people like me.

He went on to explain that he was now living in Chester and that I should visit him sometime, as he'd love to show me the sights. Bingo, Bango, Result! Right there, he'd practically asked me for a date. I was delirious and maybe now was the time to depart, whilst I still had my dignity. I was so proud that I'd managed not to throw myself at him. I couldn't wait to tell the girls.

The Invite to Chester

Trudie

As I drove home to my very uneventful life, replaying the night's events over and over in my mind, and if I was completely truthful fantasising that the whole scenario had played out totally differently, I wondered when our paths would cross again. Let's face it, he had asked me to go over to Chester to see the sights, and as I'd left he'd mentioned some party he was throwing, so I was more than hopeful. But I'd just have to be unattainable but very attainable, if you know what I mean? Well, I didn't want to come across as too desperate and too needy. I was gonna adopt a real cool persona so as to fit in with the trendy people he hung out with.

At home I paid the babysitter. I lived with Roxanne and her 18 month old baby daughter, Olivia whom I totally adored. I prepared for bed; I removed my make-up and had every intention of being awake when Roxanne arrived home so I could hear all the news of the night's events. Obviously I was desperate to know whether she'd spoken to Lloyd again. It must have been early morning before Roxy arrived back, and I was fast asleep by this time. In the morning she regaled me with funny tales of her wild night, but there was no mention of Lloyd and I wasn't going to press the point so just let it be.

Monday was a bank holiday so Roxy and I took Olivia for a picnic to a lovely spot we know at Rivington Pike. It was a fabulously relaxing day but still there was no mention of Lloyd.

Tuesday was a pretty uneventful day at work, but had I known that the following day would change my life forever, I'd probably have paid a lot more attention to enjoying the finer points of Tuesday.

Wednesday arrived and nothing of any note occurred until just before lunchtime when my phone rang. Nothing too earth-shattering there, as it was the hotline anyway, only this time when I answered (thankfully very professionally) Lloyd's voice came back at me. At first I thought I was really losing the plot or I was hallucinating. I thought I was gonna be cool, but how desperate was this? I was hearing things. How smitten must a person be to conjure up another person's voice?

He broke into my thoughts, 'Hi, sorry to ring you at work, hope it's OK?' OK! Of course it was OK. How… what… when… I was clueless, how did he even know where I worked and how had he got the number. My direct number. I went all 'fingers and thumbs', Oh voice, please don't fail me now. After what seemed like a lifetime I managed to reply that it was fine that he'd called. FINE? It was FANTASTIC!

I was trying to concentrate on what he was saying because I didn't want to miss a thing.

"Are you doing anything this weekend?"

Who cares? Even if I was, I'd change my life to accommodate him. "No, nothing special why?" came my coolish reply.

"Well after bumping into you on Sunday I was hoping that you would come over to Chester this Saturday and I'd show you those sights. I'm nothing if not consistent, I promised to show you and I'm free this weekend, so if you're free too let's make it a date".

A date? Did he say date? Too right I'm free, I'm free as a bird, I've never been so free in my entire life.

"I'd love it". An understatement if ever I'd made one.

"OK, do you know Chester at all?" And with that he imparted the directions right to his flat. No Tom Toms in those days. I was never going to forget this day for as long as I lived and I couldn't wait for the weekend. But that only gave me two and a half days to plan my every outfit, my hair and my makeup, I had to cover every eventuality.

At home I couldn't stop the verbal diarrhoea, and must have driven Roxy insane. Bless her though, she truly indulged me, and in true Roxy form she got carried away in the drama. She was dragging clothes out of wardrobes and putting together the most exquisite outfits with bags and shoes, not to mention belts. There were perfumes and body lotions and all manner of potions. Then there was the make-up, which obviously we needed to practice as there was a definite art in the application of day to night make-up in the stroke of a brush. I pretty much had it all covered but the bedroom was a bombsite and I'd have needed a 4x4 in order to ship my belongings over! Mmm, we'd just have to scale it down. This took the best part of six months, or so it felt, but eventually it all came together like a military operation and I was set and as ready as I'd ever be. All I needed now was Saturday to arrive.

The Invite to Chester 37

Chester

Trudie:

I was due at Lloyd's around 6pm; he was to finish work early. There were no mobile phones back then so as Roxy and Olivia waved me off I just knew that this was it. The journey passed in a blur and luckily I'd memorised the directions, so I just let my mind go bananas with the anticipation of what lay ahead.

I pulled up outside Lloyd's flat without a hitch other than the fact that Chester had an amazingly complicated one-way system and there were double yellow lines running along the road that the flat was on. I parked on them anyway. Well I couldn't just keep driving as I'd be sure to get lost. Lloyd had only given me directions straight to his flat, and omitted to mention where I should park. So I sat there with my eyes firmly on the rear-view mirror, looking out - not only for Lloyd, but also any predatory, over-zealous traffic wardens that may be hidden, ready to pounce and produce the final ticket of the week. Well, I'd be ready.

I spotted Lloyd in the distance, walking towards me, just exiting the city walls. He had a confident spring-like walk and he a huge grin on his face. As he approached the car he opened the passenger door. "Find it alright?" he beamed.

And that was where it began all those years ago. Needless to say it was a weekend that fairytales were made of. We were both very relaxed around each other; Lloyd really put me at my ease and gave me a confidence I never knew I had. And I realised when I left him, albeit a day or two later than I'd expected, I just knew I was totally in love with this beautiful, funny, kind, considerate, intelligent, generous, sexy man. So dreams really did come true, and I had reached my destination.

The only concern I harboured was that he had mentioned he was to leave for Aberdeen in four or five weeks' time, hence the leaving party he was throwing. I wondered how I could cram a lifetime into just four weeks. I just had to find a way. All I knew was, I wasn't going to waste a minute and I certainly wasn't going to get all stressed out and worry about it. I'm a great believer in what will be will be. C'est la vie, my friend.

Lloyd was really excited about Aberdeen and was busying himself packing and sorting and planning this huge party of his. Apparently he was quite the entertainer, always arranging events and taking people on different adventures. He'd arrange a night at the races or the dogs or plan a trip to a premiership football match for forty-plus people. He loved getting his teeth into a project and he was meticulous with the details, making sure everyone had a ball, leaving no stone unturned.

But even though he was busy he was always attentive of me and my feelings and always knew what to say or do. I began to really enjoy helping him with all his arrangements. This was something quite alien to me, as I'd never had the confidence before to throw a party or be in the limelight. I much preferred being part of the crowd and mingling, as opposed to taking centre-stage. But this giant personality of a man had started to rub off on me and I was having a fine time taking on the role of organizer. We made quite a team, even back in those days.

The night of the farewell party came round far too quickly and I'd spent much of the last month travelling to and from Chester on a daily basis, as we just couldn't get enough of each other. I'd promised him that I would definitely come and visit him in Aberdeen when he'd settled and proffered me an invite but the last thing I wanted was to be a nuisance and in the way. I loved him so much by this time that I wanted him to be happy in his new life, even if that meant I had to forfeit any dreams of 'us' that I'd fostered along the way. How could I complain? I'd had at least five weeks of pure Lloyd and that would take me through a lifetime, surely. They say it's better to have loved and lost than never to have loved at all, and at that moment in my life I knew exactly what it meant.

Roxanne looked fabulous all dressed up, so sexy, so confident and so full of fun and mischief. She was going to enjoy this party. After all she was the party animal. We were both excited as we drove to Chester that Saturday, itching to get partying.

On arrival we helped Lloyd put the nibbles out and get the flat in party mode. He was introducing us to the most technical sound system I'd ever seen in a flat, and already the tunes were thumping. Good job everyone who lived in the block had been invited or there'd be some serious complaints, I can tell you. When we were sure that all the finishing touches were in place we headed into town, where Lloyd had arranged to meet everyone.

Nights like these are what living is all about. The crowd was friendly and there was a definite magic in the air. We circulated and on occasion drifted apart but our eyes would always make contact and flirt. He would brush my hand or kiss my cheek or neck on passing by to talk with everyone there. He was without doubt the host with the most; he made everyone feel important, and gave people the time of day but never forgot to show me my worth. So for this night I knew he was mine and I was going to drink in every second of it.

Back at the flat, with music at full belt, I managed to get one or two dances with Lloyd and didn't mind when the pretty people dragged him off to talk or dance. I was totally lost in the moment and wanted the night to go on forever. At one point Lloyd mentioned that he'd booked us into a hotel and as soon as I felt like going I was to just give him 'the nod' and we could make our excuses and exit, leaving the party people behind doing what they do best - partying. Adam had made a beeline for Roxanne and there was some major flirting taking place there.

I mentioned to Roxy that at some later stage Lloyd and I were to leave and spend the last few hours alone at a hotel so we could say goodbye properly in peace and quiet, and she was more than happy about this and just wanted to carrying on 'getting on down'. I'll bet by the end of that night Roxy would have known more about Lloyd's friends than Lloyd, she could really work a room and make friends with anybody.

Just then there was a knocking, but it wasn't coming from the front door so we turned the music down to listen. There it was again, and it was coming from the window. This was somewhat bizarre as Lloyd lived in the top flat, at least four storeys high. Lloyd made his way over to the window to investigate. He slid it open and to everyone's surprise some random guy asked if he could join the party. Good Lord, he must have extremely long legs, or maybe he was a magician. How on earth was he talking at a fourth storey window? That was mighty strong wine we were drinking. Maybe he was a relative of Spiderman or Superman. Unfortunately it turned out to be somewhat less interesting. The Landlord was in the process of decorating the exterior and the passer-by had rather foolishly climbed up the scaffolding, having heard the music. Lloyd was suitably impressed that he'd gone to so much effort to gain entry when lets face it he could have just knocked at the front door!

The night was full of strange moments like that.

The Meet
(Part 2)

Lloyd:

It was late afternoon one summer-Sunday in 1984 and a sequence of events were about to unfold over the coming days that would change my life for ever.

I was living and working in Chester at the time, 24 years old and manager of a large fashion retail store. I had an apartment just outside the City walls, lots of spare cash and an endless list of clubs, bars and parties to attend.

The people I hung around with at that time were a mix of current work mates and a posse of guys and girls from Bolton who I had stayed in touch with over the years, having been born and brought up there.

I used to throw parties quite often and was planning one now, only there was a real reason for this one. It was not just the usual excuse to get leathered and keep the whole building awake into the early hours with thumping music. There was a genuine reason for this party; it was my 'leaving do'.

The company I worked for was opening new stores around the UK and I had worked in many towns and cities over the years, overseeing the shop openings. I had been asked to manage the opening of the new store in Aberdeen and even after consulting a map of Great Britain and realising Aberdeen was actually closer to Scandinavia than it was to Chester, I said yes. I managed to secure myself a huge pay rise into the bargain as the company were struggling to find anyone local with the right sort of experience for the job.

The Meet (Part 2)   45

'Aberdeen'? You must be mad! What the hell's up there?' was the standard reply as I rang round, making invites to my 'leaving do'. I had no idea what was up there except for the fact that it was the mid eighties and Aberdeen was experiencing 'boom time' off the back of the North Sea oil industry, and that was part of the attraction. Yes, I was having a good time in Chester. I loved my job, had loads of mates, and girlfriends came and went, but all my relationships at that time were pretty casual. In short there was nothing to keep me in Chester and I had a sense of adventure about me that was saying, 'Go to Aberdeen. It could be the start of a whole new life'.

My brother Adam wasn't surprised I was moving to the other end of the land. He knows me better than most and was hardly surprised that I was upping sticks again. He was more interested in the party, and in particular which and how many girls I was inviting?

"Hey, if you meet us at Cassinnellis tonight we can talk about it more," he said. He and ten or so of the Bolton Posse were going to a club near Wigan we had frequented over the years so I arranged to meet them there that evening. I called my best mate at the time Ant, and he was well up for a night out, as ever.

The party was in fact going to be a 'double leaving do' because as well as being my best mate; Ant was also my assistant manager and was making the move with me.

Ant called round to my place half an hour or so later and we had a couple of drinks while listening to some tunes, and I went through my usual routine of picking the clothes I would wear as we got into 'Club mode'. I have a real passion for clothes and always made the most of the staff discounts offered by my work. I enjoy looking good and can never understand people who just don't make the effort with their appearance. To me looking good is feeling good.

We then hit town early evening for a few more drinks before jumping in a taxi to head out to Cassinnellis, as I had arranged to meet the guys and girls from Bolton around 9 o'clock.

There was a great feel to the place that night. It was one of those evenings that follows a long hot sunny afternoon, and no one was working the next day as it was a Bank Holiday. The girls were showing off their suntans while the boys, myself included, needed little encouragement to ogle, I mean admire them. In those days it was the norm for the girls to wear very revealing outfits and this evening was no exception.

The DJ was spot on, playing all the top tunes, and the drinks were going down nicely.

The Bolton Crew were out in force and looking the business as usual, and it was as if the sunny Bank Holiday had encouraged the world and his dog to come out that evening. I bumped into many a party face I had not seen for ages.

We took over a corner of the club, strategically placed within easy reach of the three essential elements of a cracking night out, namely dance floor, bar and loos. The atmosphere was electric.

Word soon got round about my forthcoming 'leaving do' and everyone was up for it. There was some concern over who would be throwing future parties while I was living in Scandinavia, but now was not the time to be worrying about stuff like that. In any case I would be coming back at some stage, as I always did.

When I go out it's with the pure intention of having fun. I love my music and actually gigged a couple of clubs around Chester as a DJ at that time, and it was a real buzz.

I enjoy a drink, but never to the point of being completely blotto, because for me a great part of a really good night is having the memories to look back on in later years.

I've never been a guy who goes out 'on the pull'. As I say the agenda is to have a real cracking night out and if the lady of the moment happens to cross my 'party path' then I'll certainly explore the possibilities. It may sound like a pretty laid back approach to meeting women, but it's always served me well.

I can never understand guys who go out purely to 'pull a bird'. To me it sounds like too much effort. I actually know one guy who described the art of pulling purely as a 'numbers game'. He would trawl around a club asking any girl if she wanted to dance, have a drink and so on, and accept every rejection as being one step closer to the girl who would say yes.

I don't know if it ever dawned on him that the reason he was usually successful was because it was nearing the end of the night, and girls like boys wear 'beer goggles' and lower their standards as the alcohol takes control.

As I said earlier, events were about to change my life and the first of those events was about to take place as I stood at the side of the dance floor, cooling down with a bottle of Bud after a good dance session.

I was surveying the whole scene and taking in the atmosphere. I watched my mates having a great time and was thinking how they would just carry on partying into the future while I was away in Aberdeen. I wondered how often I would come home to see everyone, then quickly answered my own question: Probably not very often. That's what I am like, loads of mates, loads of great times but very few people in this world get really close to me. It may seem strange to many people but that's the way I am, even today. If you fall into the small group of people in my life who I love then you are getting it 200%, and there is nothing I would not do for the loves of my life.

Suddenly my casual observation of the partying people was focused on one person in particular. Tiny frame, a size 8 I rightly guessed, big hair, long back combed dark mane, great legs on high heels, healthy looking tan and wow, those shorts were short!

I was more than a little interested and I had not even seen the lady's face when she suddenly turned round and looked right at me. "Lloyd, I've not seen you for ages," were the words I could make out over the music as she moved towards me.

The Meet (Part 2)   49

"Hi Trudie," I responded as my mind flashed way back into the past. I had not seen her for about five years or so. We used to be 'Dance Buddies' on the club circuit. I remembered she had a fella at the time and I was 'going steady' too, but we always spent time together when we met up on nights out. Nothing more than a chat and a dance, although we once held hands as I led the way off the Dance floor at 'Clouds' in Preston one Saturday night.

Trudie was telling me a story of how she was not meant to be there that night and was going home soon, but I wasn't really listening. I was too busy being smitten, "Where's your boyfriend?", I interrupted. "There is no boyfriend". Kerching! Right answer, I thought. My mind was working at a furious rate. The situation as I saw it was this: I was looking into the eyes of this gorgeous vision from my past, where we both had wondered years ago what if we were both single? She had stepped back into my life out of the blue and I could sense was feeling the same emotions as I was that very moment. She was about to leave the club very shortly and I was moving to Scandinavia in about four weeks. I had to act quickly.

"I'm having a party in a couple of weeks will you come?" I blurted out…

Aberdeen

Trudie:

As I stood waving him off I couldn't help having this desperate lonely feeling of abandonment. Of course I was smiling, understatement, I was grinning like a Cheshire cat, because that's what you're supposed to do. You're supposed to be strong and supportive and I remember reading somewhere that if you loved someone, really loved someone, then you should let them go and if they came back then they were yours to keep. So I stood strong, blowing kisses, giving him the 'I Love You' sign as he drove away. Yes I stood strong as he went off to his new exciting life, his glamorous adventure in a land far away.

I remember reliving and cherishing every single moment of our time together and thinking that if this was the end, then that would just be tragic. How on earth would I survive 'the end'? The love I felt for Lloyd was pure, it was real, it had depth, it wasn't like the usual competitive relationships I'd experienced before, or I'd talked about with my friends, where the conclusion had always been that men really were from Mars! This was a grown-up love and it was full of magical surprises. I remember Lloyd saying 'it was electric'! That just blew me away, I was electric, wow! I knew he must have felt the same, it couldn't possibly have been all an act and if it was, what was it for? I mean I pretty much had sex with him on the first date, actually lots of sex that whole weekend in Chester, the weekend where he was supposed to be showing me the sights! So why would he have strung me along? Only time would tell.

Roxanne poured some wine. She didn't say much she just gave me a squeeze and a glass of red. I felt awful. I couldn't eat the lovely meal she'd produced and I wasn't really listening to anything she was saying. I was just existing zombie like. I had to pull myself together, I had work tomorrow and I couldn't perform like this or I'd end up joining the dole queue. Roxy suggested a night out but how could I tell her I'd never be able to go out again in case I missed his precious call? How could I spend the rest of my life this miserable? I was sure to lose all my dear friends, I mean, who in their right mind would want to spend time with a moper like me? Right bundle of laughs!

Roxy came running into the lounge, "Guess who's on the phone?" She was beaming. I immediately bolted into the hallway, no walk-around phones in those days, and in my haste I severely stubbed my toe on the lounge door, 'bugger'.

"Hello", I managed, fortunately without squealing my delight into the mouthpiece causing severe damage to his unsuspecting eardrum. My poor toe throbbed on.

"Hi, sweet cheeks", came his bright and breezy reply. It felt like he'd been gone a lifetime not the 2½ hours it had actually been. I missed him so much. "What're you doing this weekend?" his voice was like chocolate, dark and mysterious all warm and inviting with a hint of naughty thrown in. Déjà vu I thought, something about the way he said it reminded me of the Wednesday he rang me from Chester all those weeks ago, well a whole lifetime ago.

"Nothing", I managed. I wasn't usually a woman of so few words but I was in severe shock from his call, and severe toe pain to boot, and I just couldn't function, I couldn't function at all, I couldn't think straight. "How'd you fancy coming to Aberdeen and I'll show you the sights?"

What a difference 12 small words could make. I couldn't have cared less that he didn't even know the sights of Aberdeen, let alone tour guide for someone. All I knew, right there and then, was that I was ridiculously head-over-heels in love, and in lust, with the most perfect human being God decided to create and I was giddy with excitement. I was going to Aberdeen next weekend to spend time with the love of my life. Which way's Scotland?

I returned to Roxanne a different person. "Some phone call!" she teased, "Must get myself one of those, in fact the NHS should prescribe a phone like that, they'd save a fortune on Prozac". We both laughed and went onto finish that bottle of red.

I loved feeling upbeat, well who doesn't? I also loved having something to look forward to, I loved this 'being in love', unpredictable as it was the overall euphoria of being in love, this much in love, was mind-blowing.

Just like my initial trip to Chester, Roxy put together an array of outfits which again required whittling down immensely. After all, I was only spending two nights and one whole day there and if truth be known there wasn't any need for clothes at all.

I spent the week checking out maps and asking advice, this was long before the luxuries of satellite navigation, all I knew was I had to find the M74 which was somewhere at the end of the M6 going 'that' way. I had an old banger of a Ford Fiesta, 'T' reg. first time round, though in all fairness it was heavily disguised as an XR2i so I'd be fine. I was such a fake I just didn't know it. As far as I was concerned it was a pretty girly car and that was why I bought it, its wheels matched its bodywork so it fit my criteria perfectly. I wasn't interested in engines; though I'm sure Top Gear wouldn't have featured it. Fearless, that's what I was in those days, fearless and desperately in love. I'd do whatever it took to get to Aberdeen or the Moon or wherever else Lloyd decided to lay his hat (that would be my home) - I do believe someone made a song out of that!

I had butterflies in my stomach all day on Friday. I was unaware of the length of journey I was about to undertake. I'd driven to London on occasion in the past I therefore put Aberdeen on a par with London with maybe a couple of extra miles added on. It'd be a cinch, a breeze, a walk in the park. I left work early, 4pm; I wasn't even going home I was heading for Scotland straight from work. Come on Ceddie let's do it! Ceddie was short for Cedric the name I'd given my car. I liked naming inanimate objects. I gave everything a name, by labelling my stuff I felt as though I was dishing out personalities. I know it's kind of sad but I liked things like that. I was a simple soul.

Me and Ceddie set off, Aberdeenshire here we come. First step M6 no problems there. Cedric didn't have a sound system so I had my trusty ghetto blaster sat on the passenger seat playing my favourite tunes. So far so good. 6.25pm no end to the M6 yet and I'd been travelling at the national speed limit. Eventually the M6 ran into the M74, brilliant I must almost be there. I made up my mind to stop at the next services, you know stretch my legs and have a cup of tea maybe make a call to Lloyd and give him a progress report.

I can remember my bladder was almost at exploding point when the sign indicating the Welcome Break Gretna Green came into view! Gretna Green, how romantic, was it an omen? Ever the romantic I was always looking for life's clues as to what the future held in store for me. Let's face it; if this was a sign then I'd soon be married. It was strange, I'd never wanted to marry any of my previous boyfriends although I'd had proposals and I always felt dreadful when I ever so politely declined. But since I'd hooked up with Lloyd, all I could think about was being his wife. I tingled all over when I allowed myself to get carried away with such dreams.

I spent my penny, purchased the necessary provisions for sustenance and I then rang Lloyd. He answered immediately. Nice. This was definitely a good sign. I took him through my, as yet, very uneventful journey and explained exactly where I was. According to Lloyd I wasn't even halfway! Adrenalin, God bless adrenalin, at least when you're in a new relationship you have plenty of adrenalin pumping around the old system keeping you going. 'Oh well!' I thought, 'better get my skates on'.

I pointed Ceddie in the direction of the M74 and hit the gas. We sped off at break neck speed, sod the national speed limit, I had to get there as soon as I could, all this travelling is just wasted time. So music blasting and foot flat to the floor I somehow managed to attract the attention of the law. It was the first time I'd ever been a criminal and it was one of the most frightening experiences of my life. First I noticed the flashing blue lights and the stop sign. Bloody Hell it was me they were pulling over. I immediately pulled onto the hard shoulder with a million thoughts rushing through my mind, but I wasn't quite sure what to do next. Did I alight with my hands raised or did I remain in my vehicle? There must have been an etiquette, but I was unaware of procedures. I saw the Officer step out of his vehicle and I noticed he was writing something in his notebook, probably my registration number. I wound my window down as he approached, "Have you any idea what speed you were travelling at?" I could feel my bottom lip quiver; officialdom scared the life out of me. "I'm so sorry", was all I managed. I was well aware that I was travelling over the national speed limit, or was I? What was the speed limit in Scotland? Maybe it was higher. But then again maybe it was 50. I hadn't done my homework very well.

He asked me to leave my vehicle, and I dutifully obeyed. After securing Ceddie I followed in his wake to the stationary Police car. I then climbed into the rear seat. His colleague was sat in the drivers' seat. He didn't say a word as I entered the vehicle. The Officer decided to give me a breathalyser. I'd never had a breath test before. Were they going to put handcuffs on me? Were they going to take me to the station? He explained the procedure and I did exactly as he asked. I kept slowly blowing waiting for him to give me the sign to stop. At this point I must say, if you ever have the great misfortune to undergo a roadside breath test, you must blow really really slowly otherwise you'll run out of breath, as I did! Take two! My mouth was dry, my hands were shaking, my body was all a quiver and not in a nice way. Take two was just about to happen. I placed the straw in my mouth, I don't even know why I was so nervous I hadn't been drinking, I hadn't taken any drugs my only crime was the fact I may have been going a tad too fast.

Hurray, test over and I passed with flying colours. My brush with the law was also over and the nice Officer took the decision to give me a stern talking to but decided I wasn't to be thrown in the slammer, this time.

I was therefore allowed to go, but only after I'd talked them through my safe re-entry onto the motorway. Me and Ceddie skulked off all forlorn with me constantly checking my speedo.

I soon put my experience behind me as Patrice Rushen belted out 'forget-me-not' to which I merrily screeched along. I was so glad I'd bought my ghetto blaster it would have been an unbearable journey in the silence, I just prayed the batteries held out.

And the journey went on but luckily the music got better 'and the beat goes on', the Whispers were now crooning away with a little help from me. My behind was numb and I had cramp in my legs, I kept swapping my hands on the steering wheel, I must stop for another break, I'd already unfastened my rather tight therefore ever so sexy jeans to release the pressure on my bladder and now there was only one thing left I could do, and that was find a toilet and find one quick.

Oh how I wished I'd listened in geography. I glanced around and the sign in the distance indicated Perthshire, bloody hell it's no wonder this journey's taking forever I've only gone and made it to Australia! I pulled over into the Service Station, quick loo stop and then must ring Lloyd. He found my blonde moment rather amusing but explained that I was still nowhere near. Flippin heck, it just wasn't funny anymore I was even getting travel belly, not good, certainly not sexy, all swollen and dying for a trump - very lady like. Well onwards and upwards as they say, and no pain no gain, I was running through all the famous quotes to myself, distance makes the heart grow fonder. What tosh.

I climbed back in Ceddie, turned on the engine, then the ghetto blaster. Now, I know I mentioned it earlier but I do feel the need to reiterate the sentiment, God Bless the music box. I perked up immediately to the sexy sound of Rose Royce 'Magic Touch', I let it massaged my eardrums. I loved that song, it was written for Lloyd, 'You stroke me till my body's weak...' that was it. That was all I needed. Those few very naughty words and I was all fired up again. I revved Ceddie and he let out his usual meaty response, 'come on Cedric old boy, we can jolly well do this'. My foot hit the accelerator, my voice tried desperately to hit the high notes, and we were once again Aberdeen bound with spirits high.

This time I managed to stick to the speed limit which, as I'd found out, was 70 after all. I'd been driving now for over six hours and the road was poker straight, oh how I longed for a corner, or some scenery, I just wanted something else to do. My hands ached on the steering wheel. It had gone dark and I was just following my headlights. I hoped they knew the way. My stomach started churning at the thought of seeing Lloyd, I couldn't wait. I must make sure I'm looking my best. I checked the rear view mirror, 'mmm not bad'. Lippy still in place which was amazing considering all the rubbish I'd eaten and I wasn't looking too tired for once which was a real bonus. I hated that about myself, I tended to look tired without actually being tired, I never could work that out. Maybe boredom made me look tired and run down, even though this journey was tedious there was a huge prize at the end therefore I looked all lively and vibrant. I was very much liking the affect Lloyd was having on my looks.

Time went on and then I noticed my first signpost with the word Aberdeen emblazoned upon it! This really perked me up. I shuffled in my seat and took on a new driving position, at least I was going in the right direction, I must be almost there now, happy days.

The one thing I will always remember about my initial drive to Aberdeen is the fact that for about 20 miles or so, just before you hit the city, it's just straight road, then all of a sudden you see the beautiful granite buildings sprawling out before you, almost as if you're looking down onto it, it really is breathtakingly pretty and it looks so clean. I knew that nestled down there somewhere in that haven was Lloyd and I also knew he would be waiting my arrival. I drove along drinking in my new surroundings. I seemed to have been travelling through the baron desert for what seemed like a lifetime, and then came this metropolis. I felt like I'd been reborn as though I'd regained my sight. I pulled Ceddie over and studied my instructions. Crickey, I'd almost reached my destination. Well that seemed straightforward enough as the next turning on my left, by my calculation, was Union Grove. Before I pulled off, I did actually trowel more make-up on though being very careful not to achieve the Dame Edna Everage look. As I turned into Union Grove I knew his apartment was in the first big Victorian house on the left just passed the filling station.

I pulled up outside. I couldn't believe the immense size of the property then I saw the front door fly open and His Gorgeousness descend the steps, he was sporting the biggest grin and my heart was going berserk, 'Oh God please let my legs work'. He ran round to the driver's door and flung it open, his aftershave smelt divine and as always he looked delicious. I climbed out, straight into his arms, our lips met and I melted. I really had died and gone to heaven. I don't know how long we stood there and I couldn't have cared who was watching. It didn't matter how inappropriate it must have looked because as far as I was concerned the world and that moment belonged to the both of us. Magical.

Lloyd carried my bag into the apartment, merrily chatting away, and as I entered I drank in the stunning features. It was bursting full of character and it was absolutely enormous. There were the obligatory two bedrooms, a galley kitchen, bathroom, massive lounge with a weapon of a window at one end. I don't think I've ever seen such a large expanse of glass. His place was just perfect, "Good choice". "Glad you approve", came his response and we beamed at each other. I was already dreading leaving him on Sunday but I just knew I'd be back the following weekend, journey, what journey? Like I said earlier, 'piece of cake'.

Lloyd was unfortunately due in work the following day but he very thoughtfully left me sleeping to enable me to recover properly from my long journey in order that I could really enjoy the evening he'd planned. We were to meet with friends on Saturday night for drinks. Some I already knew, the guys who'd followed him up there from Chester. Others would need introduction, the new people he'd acquainted. So I undertook a rather leisurely day which included a luxurious soak in a beautiful bubble bath yummy. I got ready slowly, choosing very carefully my outfit for that evening as I wanted to wow him. I also managed to find time to make a lovely friend out of his neighbour Mrs Lott. She was 90 and the sweetest wee dot of a woman you could hope to meet. Her strong Aberdonian accent phased me somewhat but we managed with sign language and we laughed and laughed and drank lots of tea. I don't think she understood a word I said but nevertheless we gave each other huge hugs as I departed and I remember thinking that someday we could get into all sorts of mischief.

I heard the key in the door. I quickly checked the mirror. As he entered the room he let out a wolf whistle and made me spin round. He was afraid to touch me as he didn't want to spoil the effect. Oh what the heck. I ran into his arms and wished that he hadn't arranged the night out as I would have preferred a night in.

It turned out to be a bumper packed night full of merriment. Everyone made me so welcome, I felt I belonged. Now I really was fearing Sunday. We danced the night away in a Club called 'Mr G's' though we made our excuses just after midnight in order that we could have some 'us' time back at the apartment. And boy that was some 'us' time, I will never forget that first weekend in Scotland.

Needless to say Aberdeen became my weekend retreat and I became accustomed to that laborious journey. Every time I saw Lloyd I fell more deeply in love, he had the biggest eyes and his lashes were fabulous. I would say his eyes were by far his sexiest feature. Whenever I was with him I would notice something new. And he would fascinate me for hours, regaling me with tales of his youth. He had spent about five years living in Jamaica as a small child but he remembers everything. His Gran, Miss Enid (as she was known) lived in Montego Bay her house actually looked out over the bay. How romantic. How lucky to have travelled so much and to have lived in such a beautiful part of the world. I learned so much from this great man and I hated being apart from him.

So great was my desire to spend time with Lloyd that I would often call unexpectedly and he was always very grateful for my effort. I mean, 330 miles just for a brew a quick chat then back in the car. On one such occasion I couldn't gain entry into the apartment so I sat in the car outside, that was until Mrs Lott caught sight of me. She invited me in for tea and biscuits to wait in the warm. She decided to pull Lloyd's leg on his return from work and when she heard him on the stairs she went out into the hallway.

"Now listen hear young man", I heard her stern Scottish voice, "The next time you have something delivered you need to make sure that there's someone in to receive it. I'm an old frail woman and I can't lift something that large".

"I'm so sorry", cut in his apology, "But I can assure you Mrs Lott I haven't ordered anything, are you sure it's for me?"

"Oh! Quite sure. Anyway I'm not lifting it again so you'd better put your bag down and come and help me. Your delivery is taking up the whole of my living room".

She entered the room first. She winked and grinned cheekily. Lloyd dutifully followed. He could hardly believe his eyes. He took a double take then he bounced across the room and scooped me up in his arms. We all laughed and we all three danced around Mrs Lott's lounge, even dear old Mrs Lott was high on life, it was a happy happy moment and one I'll never forget. He was kissing me then he would kiss Mrs Lott and she giggled. "Now then you two youngsters, you don't want to be wasting time with an old lady, be gone with you and do whatever you do when your alone" again she gave me a cheeky wink. From that day on we three became amigos', it was an unbreakable bond and I often think of her all these years later.

The Journey

Lloyd:

There was a lot for me to contemplate so I was contemplating furiously, trying to make sense of my life and where all of a sudden it was heading. When my employers had asked me to move to Aberdeen it was an easy decision to say 'yes'. There was as ever nothing holding me back, 'nothing to lose and everything to gain' was one of my mottos at that time.

Now for the first time in a situation like this there was a hitch, no that's the wrong word. For the first time ever, there was a reason for me to stay put! Or was I being premature in my thought process? After all it had been no more than a chance meeting in a night club. We had spoken for no more that 20 minutes and then I had made the final arrangements for Trudie to come to my party via her best mate Roxanne after Trudie had vanished Cinderella like into the night.

Roxanne seemed like a really good mate. She had jumped at the chance to come to my party promising to bring Trudie with her. It turns out Trudie was living at Roxanne's following the split from her ex and Roxy gave me their home number and Trudie's works number.

How could I be contemplating not moving to Scotland based on a 20 minute blast from the past? I had invited Trudie to a party that was still four weeks away then I was going to leave for Aberdeen the next day. What sort of planning was that?! I needed to be a bit more decisive, why wait four weeks? I needed to pick up the phone and call her.

It was Wednesday morning so I figured Trudie would be at work. I therefore rang her direct number as supplied by Roxy. Seeing as it was her direct line, why was I so surprised when she actually answered? She was very surprised to hear my voice too. This is when I started to realise that Roxanne enjoyed playing mischief-maker as she had not told her best mate that she had given all her contact details to some strange guy in a nightclub the previous weekend.

So after an awkward introduction we had a great catch up and best of all Trudie agreed to come over to Chester that coming weekend. I promised to show her the sights that Saturday evening after I had finished work.

Now I really had stuff to think about. I now had four weeks to get to know my blast from the past. I needed to know if my reservations about leaving were based on anything more than that 'brief encounter', of a few days ago.

The four weeks came and went all too quickly. Trudie had come over to Chester the first weekend after we met and we got on as though we'd known each other all our lives. The original plan was for her to come over for the Saturday but we were having such a good time it was Wednesday before we recovered our senses and decided we had both better go back to work.

Then there had been the big 'leaving do'. Another great success, if we leave out the fact that it was the Police who eventually called 'time' on the merriment early on the Sunday morning. Although I suppose it served me right for bunking off to a local hotel with Trudie while leaving my brother Adam in charge. Threatening to throw my landlord down the stairs for complaining about the mess was not quite the way I would have handled things. The fact that the landlord had to negotiate his way through a number of drunken semi naked revellers had not done much to help his mood either.

My excuse of spending the night in the hotel was pretty valid in that I wanted to grab at least a few hours alone with Trudie, and I needed to sleep before tackling the long drive up to Aberdeen. Actually long drive is an understatement. It took me over eight hours to make the journey giving me lots of time to contemplate my new found relationship.

I felt very positive about how we had hit it off over the past four weeks. I could feel there was a special bond already forming between us. I was not on the lookout for a lasting relationship but I knew I wanted to be around Trudie as much as possible.

As the miles to Aberdeen rolled by, it began to seem as though my journey would never end. I started to realise that distance was going to play a major part in deciding if we stayed together or not.

We had both promised the other we would keep in touch and visit each other as often as possible. No firm rules or commitments, we were going to let love take its natural course and if we were meant to stay together long term then it would happen.

As night began to fall and I still had a couple of hours before I got to Aberdeen I started thinking of other modes of transport that could eat up the miles more efficiently than this laborious drive. The first alternative that sprung to mind was the train, yes that would be a good way to make the journey, let someone else take the strain. The next thing I thought about briefly, and I mean very briefly, was flying. I didn't give it too much consideration because I am the worlds worst when it comes to getting on aeroplanes. Why? Because it's not natural! A great big chunk of metal no matter how aerodynamic is not meant to leave the ground, particularly with me in it.

Don't get me wrong, I do fly if it's absolutely necessary. I have taken holidays abroad but believe me when I say getting there and coming back on the plane is by far the worst part of any holiday for me. I'm the same with these crazy rides that thrill seekers go on at places like Alton Towers. I don't consider risking my life on some rickety 'man-made' contraption, a thrill. Has no one ever heard of 'human error'? I don't need to get on 'The Big One' to get to work or to reach a holiday destination so consequently I have never set foot on the thing and never will.

As Trudie got to know me she realised fear of flying was my thing, and in a weird way it gave her an indication of how serious I was about our relationship.

I had been in Aberdeen a few months where during that time we had managed to see each other on quite a few weekends. Mostly Trudie had taken the long drive because she could finish work early on a Friday and head north, whereas I generally worked Saturdays. I had made the odd journey in the opposite direction by hire car or train and with a Bank Holiday coming up I was due to catch the train down to Preston to spend a long weekend. However, probably because it was a Bank Holiday weekend, the train timetables were patchy to say the least and whilst I could get a train south there was absolutely nothing coming back north when I needed it.

I rang Trudie to tell her. "You could fly?" She had offered half-heartedly, not really expecting a positive riposte. "OK, I'll go and see if there's a flight", I said while wondering in amazement who had taken control of my vocal cords! I suppose it's like going on a holiday I told myself as I headed off to the 'Flight Agents' shop. Oh, the things we do for love.

It turned out there were no planes leaving Aberdeen for Manchester when I needed one. What a relief! At least I could say I'd tried, even though I felt like the worlds biggest coward. I was about to leave when the Booking Agent started getting rather too clever and helpful for my liking. She went onto explain that there was a flight from Manchester back to Aberdeen at exactly the time I needed to come back. "OK Miss Clever Clogs, but fat lot of use that is, when you can't get me on a flight there in the first place", (I thought to myself). But she was good at her job, too bloody good. 'She could book me on a train down on the Friday afternoon and get me on the flight back on Monday'. She just had to check there were still seats available on the plane. "Oh dear, it seems to be fully booked". HA! Not so clever now are we Missy, I smiled to myself. "Oh! There's been a cancellation this morning", she said rather too excitedly for my liking, "I can give you the last seat on the plane, would you like me to book it?" No, just give me the details of the imbecile who cancelled so I can go round and set about him with a baseball bat I was thinking… and stop looking so pleased with yourself you over helpful cow!

Then the voice-jacker took over again and I could hear him using my vocal cords to agree to this life endangering journey. Then somehow my body was being controlled by an alien presence as I signed where I needed to sign my own death warrant and then to cap it all paid for the privilege!

As I left the office a condemned man my first thought was to go back in and get that woman's name and the details of her head office. I would send in a letter of complaint. Bloody over-helpful, over-zealous staff booking people onto flights of death, what the hell did she think she was doing? Then I remembered the reason for my flight of death, I was going to see Trudie again and anyway I was only going to die on the way back. It would make me enjoy my weekend even more knowing it was my last on this mortal coil.

I would let it go this time. I wouldn't report her to Head Office. I would be brave and take the flight home pretty much the way I had to when I went abroad on holiday. I began to look forward excitedly to the fantastic few days Trudie and I would spend together.

Before I knew it the fantastic few days were history and Trudie was driving me to Manchester Airport. I had tried not to make too big a deal about my fears for the flight home but she knew I was worried and while not wanting to sound like a big baby I was fearing flying alone for the first ever time! Who was going to hold my hand particularly at the point that scared me most, the take off? When the plane thunders down the runway at breakneck speed before defying the laws of gravity to take off, when I feel like jumping out of my seat and screaming at the cabin crew to let me get off. Who was going to hold me down and stop me from doing it this time?

"You'll be fine", Trudie assured me. "You'll be there before you know it. Aberdeen won't seem so far away by plane". 'Easy for you to say', I thought. Trudie loves flying and going on Big Dippers and other wild rides, there was no way she could understand my fear. Much the same way I could never understand her fear of spiders. If you don't share someone's phobia you can't appreciate what all the fuss is about.

We found the check-in desk and that's when I first started to suspect that all was not as it seemed. The check-in clerk told me my hand luggage was too big and would therefore have to be checked-in, to go in the hold of the plane! Too big? It was only a sports bag! We said our goodbye's and I made my way to

Gate No. 16 as per my flight instructions and that's where my suspicions started to turn to paranoia. I distinctly remember 'Miss Clever Clogs' in Aberdeen telling me she had managed to book me on the last remaining seat on this plane, so why was there just me and about ten other blokes waiting for the aircraft at Gate No. 16?

Then I got my answer. Surely someone was having a laugh at my expense. The jalopy that taxied onto the tarmac in front of Gate No. 16 was not fit to be a fairground ride let alone actually take off with people in it and fly to Aberdeen. That's why my bag had to go in the hold, that's why there were just a dozen or so passengers! The plane was so small I would probably have to sit on someone's lap. It had bloody propellers and they looked ill-fitted! I had managed to get quite a good deal on the travel tickets I bought even though it was a Bank Holiday weekend and now I was beginning to understand why. I was going 'crop-spraying'! I was flying home in a plane not much bigger than a two-seater crop-sprayer!

Panic was setting in! I looked back at the main building of the Airport to see if I could spot Trudie but who was I kidding, she would be well on her way by now. She knew I was going on an 'Air-fix' plane and was, by now, making good her escape.

This time when the alien presence took control of my body I was grateful because it walked me down the steps to the tarmac when my natural instinct was to turn tail and run back into the airport.

The alien then climbed the rickety little steps on to the plane using my legs before sitting me down in the tiniest of seats directly above the left wing and just behind the dodgiest looking of the two propellers.

This was not really happening to me was it? I imagined what it must be like for those people you hear about who go into surgery for an operation but the anaesthetic doesn't knock them out to proper effect, and they are awake throughout the whole operation but unable to speak. Unable to protest about the distress they are experiencing. Yes, I was having my very own 'triple bypass surgery' without anaesthetic. I was experiencing what for me, was a living nightmare and the worst was yet to come.

My stress levels were going through the roof and as yet the plane hadn't even moved, thank goodness for small mercies but it was not to be for very long.

I looked round the plane and started to take in my surroundings. The first thing I noticed was that even though I was in the third seat back out of six, I was practically looking over the pilots shoulder. I could clearly read all the dials on his instrument panel, that's how small this plane was. There was an air hostess who was busy strapping herself into a seat that was positioned right at the back of the plane, maybe she new something we should know I remember thinking as I quickly scrabbled around looking for my safety belt.

The whole proceedings took on real comedy proportions when the pilot got out of his seat to stand up, he turned round to face us as he leaned into the cabin and delivered his pre-flight spiel. He informed us that refreshments were being provided; flasks would be coming round, one of tea and one of coffee. I kid you not! I wanted to shout out 'Never mind tea and coffee, where's the bloody brandy?' I did not need a warm beverage at this time I needed strong alcohol to numb the senses, to get me through the peril that lay ahead.

All too soon it was time to go. Time to get airborne. And the crop-sprayer was being revved up. It sounded like a lawn-mower, a pretty powerful lawn-mower but a lawn-mower nonetheless. The dodgy propellers were turning, nowhere near fast enough for my piece of mind but I assumed they would speed up as required when necessary. Then we lurched into motion as we began the short trip to the runway with the windows vibrating and seats juddering, this piece of junk did not even cut it as a decent car let alone an aeroplane!

The next comedy moment came when we had to wait at a little junction at the side of the runway. We had to 'Give Way' while the 'proper' planes took off and landed. We had to stay out of the way of the real aviators before finally being granted permission to take off ourselves.

We began to trundle along the runway and under normal circumstances I would be pinned back in my seat with fear as the aircraft roars with power and impossible pace before thrusting skywards. However, these were not normal circumstances and instead I was thinking things like, 'when will the propellers actually start turning quickly?' and, 'surely a plane can't take off whilst doing just 30mph?" Don't even get me started on the sounds the damn thing was making. And still we ambled along at a pace that made 'Driving Miss Daisy' look like Burt Reynolds in 'The Cannonball Run'!

I looked into the cockpit, the pilot was no more than 7 or 8 feet away, I could dive over there and take him out, make him abort the take off and wait until he had a real plane to fly. He was clearly insane if he thought he was going to get this thing off the ground and my actions in hijacking this flight would be seen as heroic as opposed to criminal. I would be commended for saving so many lives by my brave actions against the 'madman pilot'!

Before I could put my rescue plan into operation however, I felt a strange but familiar sensation that forced me to cling onto my seat. It was the familiar, but very scary, sensation of leaving the ground. We were indeed taking off at 30mph! OK the pilot was giving it the full works and maybe we were hitting 40mph by now but the front wheels had definitely lifted from the tarmac, conclusive evidence if anyone was still in doubt, that we had a lunatic at the controls. He was trying to defy gravity and take off in a plane that was travelling at the same speed as a milk float!

I closed my eyes but opened them again a minute later on the basis that not seeing was scarier than watching the whole horror-show unfold in front of me. A lot can happen in a minute and I was surprised to see that we were actually a good way from the ground below when I looked out of the window. Just as I was starting to think things weren't as bad as I'd feared. The madman masquerading in the pilots outfit decided it was necessary to change the direction we were flying in.

Now, in a huge Boeing type aeroplane this sort of manoeuvre is no big deal even to a 'soft pants' like me... but in a motorised kite? Turning left or right is like doing a death defying 'Red Arrows' type stunt. The sky suddenly appeared to be below me while the ground was over my head. It felt as though we would all fall out of the plane at any second. My stomach began to lurch and I wondered which way my vomit would fly, down towards the ceiling or up to the floor? I decided throwing up was not a good option, it would make a horrendous mess in such close quarters and I could not entertain the idea of being sick on my clothes. I had a reputation to preserve and hint of puke was not the latest fashion trend.

I had to get a grip and the sooner the better, 'think about it Lloyd, you are up here like it or not, there's nowhere else to go for the next hour or so, get used to it. Relax, plane crashes are very rare, you have more chance of getting knocked down by a bus in the high street', etc. etc. etc. I was doing my best to recall and use every bit of logic or flying statistic that I could muster in order to bring myself down from the heightened state of panic I was experiencing and gradually found myself relaxing a little. Don't' get me wrong here, I don't mean relaxing as in 'by the pool under a sunshade with a Pina Colada' relaxing. I just relaxed enough to avoid soiling my pants or wearing hint of puke for the remainder of the journey.

At least the worst part of flying for me was over, I had survived the take-off and now there was just the landing to master then I would be back on solid ground I could do that. I had no choice in the matter but I could do it I told myself. But my bravery and commitment to love were really going to be tested on this day. I had survived an ordeal that for me and others like me who hate flying, was a living nightmare but believe it or not it still wasn't over. I must have omitted to read the small print on my travel documents or failed to hear if Miss Clever Clogs in Aberdeen had told me, but whatever the reason I swear I nearly had heart failure on the spot when about fifty minutes into the journey, at a point where I was thinking 'nearly there, we'll be landing soon and it'll all be over', the mad pilot announced over his shoulder that we would be landing in Dundee for refuelling before taking off again to complete the journey to Aberdeen!

So this crappy little aeroplane couldn't even carry enough fuel to get us all the way to Aberdeen in one go. I didn't even know Dundee had an airport!

The rest of the journey to this day remains a hazy blur as I can only assume my brain shut down in order to protect me in some weird way. I know I was there on that plane but in a strange detached third party sort of presence. I felt like I was watching from outside my body as the plane 'Red Arrowed' around and down over a bridge that crossed the river near to the airfield before landing. I watched yet another comedy moment as the pilot slid open his window and instructed the guy on the ground to "Fill her up!" Then, by the time we went through the whole ridiculous take off procedure again I just didn't care anymore. I was too far gone to care and barely remember landing in Aberdeen. I do remember how my legs seemed to be made from jelly as I finally emerged from the plane and made my way shakily down the steps and it was a good couple of days before I felt physically well again after my ordeal.

They say every cloud has a silver lining (excuse the pun) and although I could see no positives whatsoever at the time, that flight had proved to be the catalyst in me deciding that first of all, never again in my life would I set foot in a plane of that size, and secondly I was no longer prepared to be so far away from Trudie. I knew without a shadow of a doubt that I wanted to spend the rest of my days with her and soon began making plans to come home. One thing was guaranteed in that I would not be coming home by aeroplane.

The
Proposal

Trudie

My visits to Aberdeen were by now frequent to say the very least, I would undertake that laborious journey every weekend and I'd even taken to calling in for a cuppa mid week. Now some of you may consider my 'Lloyd addiction' and my actions to be somewhat crazy but I knew he felt the same way. He made me feel ten feet tall, my heart would sing permanently from the moment I opened my eyes in the morning to the minute I climbed into bed of an evening. I was truly living the dream and hoped that long may the immense feeling of euphoria continue.

Towards the end of the year Lloyd took me to Dunnottar Castle in Stonehaven. It was breathtaking. There wasn't a soul in sight and there had been a thick even snowfall. It was crisp and bright, and as the sun kissed the snow it glistened. It was very cold but ever so still. Stonehaven Castle (as I preferred to call it) stood high on the cliff-top overlooking the sea; I'd never seen anything so beautiful. We left the car and walked towards its immense structure, the snow crunching under foot and twinkling like diamonds in the sunshine. The sea wind was icy against our skin forcing us to turn-up the collars on our coats. I for one was extremely glad that I'd worn my scarf and gloves.

The castle had been shut up for the winter months, which was a shame as I'd have loved to have seen inside. I made a promise to myself to return and bask in its glory in the summer months, though to be honest; I wasn't relishing the thought of sharing this idyllic place with the tourists. It was beyond romantic there were no words to describe this dramatic cliff-top fortress.

Suddenly a figure appeared in the distance. Lloyd made towards him and I followed. He was an elderly gentleman and he was pointing towards the Castle. "Do you want to go in?" "Oh yes please", came my eager reply. He held out a huge bunch of keys on a large hoop. He began to finger through them as he made to the entrance. He reminded me of a character from a Dickens novel. He wore a long grey woollen coat which was almost too big for his frail frame. He wore the obligatory fingerless gloves. He also wore the kindest smile. I could hardly contain my excitement, how lucky were we? How did he know we were here? Where had he come from? All manner of questions were racing through my mind as he unlocked the fortress and gestured inside.

As we entered my eyes were dancing all around, I felt I shouldn't walk on the newly laid snow for fear of tarnishing its perfection. Lloyd left me standing there drinking in the glory. When he returned he took me round the castle and told me the story surrounding it. I was enthralled. He was so knowledgeable; he'd obviously done his homework. We stood at the very top, looking down on to the sea below. The sun was high in the sky as he turned to me and proffered a glass. Where had the glass come from? And what was in it? Champagne! Why?

Lloyd slowly turned towards me and began, "I have waited all my life to meet someone so perfect, someone who makes me feel the way I do now, someone who doesn't control or judge, someone who is so genuine, kind and loving, someone who makes me laugh and doesn't look for any negatives. You always find the positives and I can't bear to think of my life without you in it. You have given me so much in such a short period of time. You believe in me more than I do myself. I love you with all my being and I want you to think seriously before answering this question, would you do me the honour. would you be my wife?"

I could not believe my ears, the man of my dreams chose me! By now Lloyd had gone down on one knee and he produced the most exquisite diamond ring I think I have ever seen. Tears were blurring my vision and I reached out and touched his cheek, "I have wondered all my life if I would find true love. And if I did, would my true love recognize and truly love me, but I could never in my wildest dreams have predicted such a romantic setting or a more perfect proposal. I would be honoured to be your wife and I would be honoured to share your life. Yes I'll marry you Lloyd Thompson and I'll love you till the day I die". I didn't need time to think, I'd known from the first moment I'd set eyes on Lloyd when I was just 16 years of age. Some things you just know for sure.

Peoples' Insensitivities

Lloyd:

'So whose fault is it that you can't get pregnant?' What a ridiculous question to ask two people who are putting their whole lives on hold in an effort to produce offspring. However this was a question often put to us by 'well meaning friends' who obviously had not thought about what they were really saying. 'Whose fault is it', suggests that one of you is purposely doing something wrong in order to hinder the process. And if as a couple you are unprepared for this quite common intrusion into your situation, then the consequences could be far reaching. We know many couples who have not managed to stay the course and have been driven apart by the stresses and strains of trying to start a family. You have to stand firm as a unit and support each other every-step of the way in order to survive what, to many, will be the hardest challenge they'll ever face in life.

Our answer would always be the same, 'It's no one's fault!' We were in this together and Mother Nature was not being quite as cooperative as she might be. Unless you have personally experienced infertility you can never really know the pain and anguish suffered by those like ourselves, unfortunate enough to be in that situation.

To me the weirdest thing about our whole time of being childless was the fact that we were never in a position to really say, 'we cannot have children'. Because while the birth of a baby is conclusive proof that yes you can have children, for us and I'm sure many others like us, there was never any concrete evidence that we were without doubt incapable of producing offspring. In a strange way that would be a lot easier to deal with. Immediately tragic, but in the long run at least there would be a tangible fact that we could in the first instance acknowledge then gradually learn to accept, before moving on with our lives.

It's the not knowing that makes the whole infertility thing so very hard to deal with. Not knowing if it's best to just push on with your career. Not knowing how your lives will be stacking up this time next year. Not knowing if you will need to find a few thousand pounds to fund another IVF treatment. Not knowing if trying to adopt a baby would be the best course of action to take. Not knowing when the pain and yearning in your heart will stop.

There is the most gut-wrenching and unique feeling of loss each month that goes by. Some people may say, 'how do you have a feeling of loss for someone who has never existed?' But you do. That's why every case of infertility is so unique and personal to the individual couples that it affects.

As dramatic as it sounds every month that you realise that once again you have failed to conceive, feels like a bereavement.

There are varying levels of intensity to the pain depending on how far you have come on that particular cycle. I suppose I am saying that the hurt is bad enough when you try by conventional means to have a baby only to get to the end of the month and find out that once again it's not to be. Let alone going through a whole IVF treatment cycle, where you actually see the fertilised embryos sitting in a Petri dish, then magnified on a screen, before having them placed in the womb. To then carry these embryos for a period of time before losing them is most devastating.

The times we faced up to this were the times I felt absolutely useless. As a man how could I ever possibly know the emptiness that Trudie was feeling having, 'lost her babies'. And no, that's not an exaggeration it's what actually happens each time a living embryo is placed in the womb but sadly fails to cling on to life, a woman loses her baby.

As a man how could I find the right words to say to try and make things better? How could I really empathise without really ever knowing how she was physically feeling? How could I really walk the lonely miles in her shoes in order to feel her pain? Fact is I couldn't. No man can. You have to be a woman to understand the real pain of infertility. We men just have to give love and support in the best way we can without questioning any of the feelings our loved ones' are experiencing, because we can never truly know the anguish they are going through at that time.

Each month would bring new hope be it through conventional methods of trying to get pregnant or via one of the 6 failed IVF's we went through.

144 months of thinking 'yes this is the one, this time we will be pregnant' but suffering the immense

feeling of loss 144 times over those 12 years. But you have to keep bouncing back!

Not for a moment would I ever claim to be the driving force on our mission to realise our dream of having a child, Trudie was the rock on which our determination was built as over the years she led the charge and dealt with anything that was thrown in our direction. 144 times she cried until she could cry no more then each time came bouncing back stronger and more determined than before! She would administer her own drugs by injection when we were on treatment. She would get up at silly times in the morning to travel to hospital in Manchester for appointments while still holding down her full-time job. When one doctor suggested she may be getting too old for further IVF treatment he was given short shrift as Trudie told him that would be our decision to make as we were the ones paying the medical fees! This tiny little lady made me realise on an almost daily basis why I loved her so much. I was, and still am so proud of her and the way she carried us through those times.

Not that I made it easy for her all the time. In the beginning I was of the mindset that if she wanted a baby then fine by me but if nothing happens then so be it. In short, I wasn't really bothered either way. We were a young married couple with plenty of living still to do. I was 26 and Trudie 25 when we married. We had careers to push, holidays to take, loads of wild parties and clubs to go to and surely having a baby would just get in the way of this great time we were having?

I know now that in those early months and years of disappointment I should have been more supportive of Trudie instead of saying things like 'I'm not even sure I want a baby. Our life is just fine as it is!'

At one point I even got to thinking that Trudie only ever instigated sex if it was the right time of the month for getting pregnant. And my Manly insecurities would have me scanning my mental calendar in the hope that we were 'getting it on' purely because we found each other totally irresistible as we had always done. I know it sounds wet but I really hated the thought that I may be being used purely as some sort of mating stud.

I remember when we were going through one particularly tough period pointing out a random guy in the street and saying to Trudie, "If you knew for certain that guy could get you pregnant, I think you would go with him". She never answered at the time but some years later admitted that she was so consumed with the need to get pregnant that yes she probably would have!

Now as I approach my 50th birthday and our wonderful son approaches his 11th I really do believe that all the years of trying for him were for a reason.

By the time our son was born we had lived our youthful lives, been to the wild parties, had the holidays and most of all matured as people. Too often I hear of couples having babies to hold a relationship together or having kids while still only kids themselves, then the foundations for building a family unit are too weak to support the demands of life brought upon every family and ultimately the whole thing comes crashing down.

Our family unit may be small but is ever so secure and we see evidence of that everyday in our precious baby boy. Often I look at him and cast my mind back 20 odd years when I used to say, 'I'm not even sure I want a baby?' If only I knew then what I know now, parenting and the joy it brings is an honour some of us are so lucky to receive even if it takes 12 years.

Testing Our Sanity

Trudie:

I remember as a small child my Dad taking me to see Tommy Steele in 'Half a Sixpence', it was the first time I'd ever been to the theatre to see a live production. It was awe inspiring and from that very moment I was totally hooked, I fell in love with the magnitude of it all. It's a fantastic experience, a place to run and hide when life feels scary. A whole new existence that can be summoned at will.

My new found theatre addiction would prove invaluable to my sanity in my adult life so thank you Dad for the introduction.

Manchester's St Mary's Hospital is enormous and my sense of direction isn't my strongest quality. I really hoped Lloyd would be on time as I was seriously stressed. I was to meet him in the car park for our first official appointment.

We had already attended the open seminar in the Hospital's auditorium with the hordes, where we met the great man himself and he addressed every angle and every complication of the invasive procedure we were to face. Not that his frank words deterred any of us. At this stage he could have delivered a speech outlining pure and utter torture ahead and I'd have signed up for the ride as long as the end result was a baby.

There must have been over a hundred couples at that first meeting but this one was just for us and I was stressed because I was running late. It had been difficult to get away from work and then the traffic was nose to tail on and off for most of the journey. I was sweating buckets and my clammy hands were almost crushing the steering wheel with my tense grip.

I loved my position as a legal secretary but I'm one of those people who always manages to land a post where there's just far too much job. I would continually meet myself coming back and my colleagues were equally as frantic. So even though I could do my job and I enjoyed it, it was without doubt very demanding. The hassles of the job coupled to that ridiculous journey from Bolton to Manchester then add my panic of 'where's Lloyd', all amounted to an almost unbearable pressure bearing down on me. I really did feel as if I was losing my marbles.

Deep breaths I told myself and calm. Breathe in through the nose and out through the mouth, I'd heard that somewhere, so I thought I'd give it a go. 'Come on Lloyd where are you?' I got out of my car and searched the car parks, up and down I wandered remembering to breathe in and out all the while - this was easy peasy so why wasn't I feeling the benefits, why was I still so screwed up inside? Still breathing in and out all the while!

Lloyd pulled onto the car park and I pointed towards my car so he could park next to me, 'we want to be together' I thought to myself, how sad? He got out of the car. He looked amazing, very neat and tidy, you'd have thought he'd been pampering, preening and preparing himself all morning, he always looked fab.

I wouldn't say he was gifted because he was luckily born perfect, he didn't need any tweaking, whatever ensemble he chose to throw on always managed to look as though Gok Wan had played a major role. I loved and I hated this about Lloyd! Well, it was hard to match and it was even harder to compete! I must get myself Goked one day, I mused.

We strode into the Hospital hand-in-hand and made our way down the long corridors until we found the waiting room. We informed the staff of our arrival and dutifully plonked ourselves down for the inevitable laborious wait.

"Mr. and Mrs. Thompson?" We stood up immediately, having hardly touched the seats, she smiled, "This way please". We followed, she was lovely, and she chatted merrily as we followed her. I couldn't tell you what she talked about as I was too busy focusing on the butterflies in my stomach. This was it! In my mind I was already pregnant. I'd made it through every stage and now we were to embark on the most thrilling part of our journey so bring it on! I had the knowing feeling that it was already 'in the bag', as they say.

The doctor introduced herself and asked us to take a seat. The room was old, full of antique furniture, not like a Hospital room at all. She placed herself behind the huge desk. I think the room reminded me of a grand library; there were even stained glass windows and ladders attached to the shelving to enable easy access to the higher books, how divine. I clung onto Lloyd's hand; I'd lost the ability to speak due to my nerves. I noticed she was talking but I wasn't hearing. 'Come on, get a grip', I chastised myself.

"Before we can begin, I need to be sure that you're both mentally strong enough to cope with the whole procedure", she was smiling, I liked her she somehow made it feel OK to have to be certified sane! How bizarre. "So I've made an appointment for you to see the counsellor who will assess you".

EH! We came all the way here to be told we need to wait for another appointment regarding our mental health. I felt Lloyd's grip tighten, he was trying to reassure me and keep control of my fiery temper - I should have been a redhead. I had legged it out of work having started at stupid o'clock this morning in order to accommodate this appointment only to be told we had to return for another appointment at a later date with a shrink. 'You're having a laugh', I thought.

Good old Lloyd had taken control and was merrily chatting away with the doctor, whom I hasten to add I no longer liked! I had to get a grip, my mental state could seriously let me down and I wasn't about to fall at the first hurdle. I scraped myself together enough to ask her when the appointment would be. To my utter delight we were to see the counsellor straight after the meeting with the doctor, happy days, it was already booked for today, phew! I found myself warming to her again. She began to talk us through the whole process and the timescales involved. She happily answered all our questions and made sure that we were as fully versed as possible in all aspects, she paid due attention to our understanding of the procedure. She was witty and very charming which helped me relax. Once the questioning had ground to a natural halt she picked up her phone and arranged for us to be taken to see the counsellor.

Before we departed her office, she confirmed that we would meet up with her later on in the day once she'd received the counsellor's conclusions as to our suitability/stability.

I must admit this part terrified the life out of me. What would happen if they found out that I was, without a shadow of doubt, completely nutty? I mean, would they be duty bound to inform Lloyd or could we just keep him in the dark, you know, due to data protection and all? More scary though, what if Lloyd was barking and his pleasant façade was just an act cleverly disguising an axe murderer? What if they told us we weren't compatible at all in fact we actually despised the bones of each other? Well, shrinks can convince you of anything, or so I thought.

I saw them on a par with Paul McKenna, they'd put us under hypnosis then make us do all manner of foolish things whilst all the time assessing our mental state. Yup, they truly gave me the heebie geebies! I was not looking forward to this part at all.

I quietly voiced my concerns to Lloyd who at least gave them the courtesy of consideration and didn't just laugh out loud. He was very good like that he never belittled any of my fears and with hindsight I did sound more than a tad unhinged. He explained the way he saw it, the medical team were looking after our best interests and also, without sounding too callous, they were in fact ticking boxes. He went onto explain that if we cleared every stage with as near to 100% perfection as possible then the Hospital stood a better chance of success therefore hitting their targets. Cruel as this may sound, government funding requires proof of success. Fact of life. In short they were probably hand-picking their own best chance at success, therefore if they saw fit to allow us onto the programme they were in fact implying that they considered us as candidates 'more likely to succeed'.

Lloyd was always philosophical like that.

All of a sudden we'd reached our destination and were shown into the 'lab'! That was my interpretation; after all we were the lab rats, the fodder. I wondered what tests they had in store for us. I squeezed Lloyd's hand took a deep breath and entered. I couldn't have been more nervous had I been facing my own execution. This whole process was definitely making me melodramatic.

Once inside I was pleasantly surprised. The counsellor seemed extremely normal almost pleasant was her persona. She proffered tea and biscuits. My suspicious mind was off again, was this where she'd lull us into a false sense of security? I scanned the room with my beady eye looking for two-way mirrors. Oh yes I'd watched the Bond films. I bet there was a microphone attached to her jacket.

There goes the melodrama again! She actually just chatted to us, explaining all the stresses and strains that the IVF procedure could place on a relationship and the financial implications that we had to consider, she wanted to know our feelings. How did we feel about the hand we'd been dealt? We talked in length about the sadness, the anger and the frustrations. We aired many, if not all of our grievances. All-in-all it was a very pleasant hour or so and yes I have changed my views.

At this point the counsellor needed to brief the doctor so Lloyd and I went off for a nice cup of tea in the canteen. Nice cup of tea? What tosh. We went for a brew and a ginormous worry. The 'decision making' was in the lap of the Lords at this stage. We both knew that if we hadn't sold ourselves to these two people then we had no chance of being allowed a place to carry on. Oh boy I had a stomach full of knots. Part of me was excited, like a child on Christmas Eve, the other part of me couldn't stand the sickening suspense. Little did I know then that these feelings would continue to feature heavily in my life for many years to come?

The Failure

Trudie:

It was 29th January 1990 it was a Monday morning, well actually it was 4am and we were getting ready to go to Manchester St Mary's before work to collect and administer my very first injection. This was where the cycle began for real. This is the part where they start to suppress my natural cycle (put me through the change). Since being chosen to take part in the whole in vitro fertilisation process I've hardly been able to sleep with excitement so 4am was no problem to me whatsoever I couldn't wait to get up and get started.

On arrival at the hospital we hurried to the waiting room, so accustomed were we to this place now it just felt like coming home. We said a quick 'Hi' to everyone to let them know we were 'ready and able' and we were soon called into the treatment room. After a quick check on my blood pressure it was straight down to business and onto the injection.

This part I really wanted to administer myself as it would save a daily trek to Manchester or to my own doctors. In order to be allowed this honour I firstly needed to convince the Team that I would be able to inject myself. The nurse slowly showed me how to prepare the solution making sure there were no air bubbles in the syringe. Piece of cake! I was then to administer the drug into my leg without hitting any blood vessels. I placed the needle into the skin I'd pinched up and I fed it slowly along. I pulled back on the syringe head, making sure no blood appeared, when I was fully sure that I hadn't hit a blood vessel I slowly began to plunge the liquid into my leg. Whoopee Mission accomplished. I couldn't believe how well I'd done; I think Lloyd was pretty impressed too. The nurse asked if I'd be comfortable with this procedure every morning, which I obviously was, then she promptly left to collect my fortnights supply.

We, quite rightly discussed my bravery on the way home in great detail, nothing like a pat on the back! The part I was more thrilled with was the fact that I'd managed the whole process without hurting myself at all, what a huge relief that was because if I was truthful, I was petrified. I never for one moment believed that I would be able to administer an injection and to be honest, I'd never in my life had a pain free injection, so I was totally proud of me. From now on waxing would be a breeze.

On arrival at work I placed my drugs in the fridge and regaled everyone with tales of my heroics even showing the wee pinprick still visible on my leg. The whole legal firm were behind this IVF venture as no one in the Company had ever met anyone unfortunate enough to have to go through it. Well, they probably had, but in those days not many people talked about their infertility. I think this was due to the fact that they saw it as their own failing and I put this down to the pressures society places on you to procreate. Not me though I'd always been big on wearing my heart on my sleeve. I am what I am, take me or leave me, no heirs or graces here. I liked giving people something to talk about whether it be in the positive or the negative, peoples opinions didn't hold any fears for me. It wasn't always that way though because I used to place too much credence on what folk thought, I therefore found this self-confidence and self-belief one of the best aspects of ageing, it just didn't matter anymore.

I think I remember the 30th January just as vividly as the previous day due to the fact that I now had to administer this wee injection without any medical staff or help whatsoever. All I had now was the lovely Lloyd and Neil the cat! Very daunting! Lloyd's suggested method was 'do it fast' then cuddle Neil for comfort as this was one of my favourite pastimes. I remember thinking we'd better actually remove Neil as he may see it as a game and start fighting the needle, he'd fight anything. He was a big ginger tom cat and he was always confirming his supremacy within the home by way of a fight, but then after all he was an alley cat born and bread.

He was therefore removed to another room for safety reasons and Lloyd went into the kitchen to make a cup of tea. I sat watching 'Whinny the Pooh', it reminded me of my childhood. I still love Pooh bear, my favourite book being 'The House at Pooh Corner'. I sat trying to muster my enthusiasm. Yup Lloyd was right; get it over as quick as I could then I'd be able to relax with a nice brew before getting ready for work. Here goes!

Again it wasn't so bad. I should have been a nurse or doctor; I was very good at this. Two down and as yet no side affects. Again we discussed my great courage.

With each day that passed and with each injection administered came a new found confidence, I grew more and more self-assured; I was now certain that I had the ability and the personal resources to succeed. Admittedly I had started getting the odd night sweats and sometimes I would have flushes during the day. But nothing that I had endured thus far had phased me; the whole process was a lot less traumatic than the picture they had painted. I was extremely relieved and I slowly began to be more upbeat and positive about the whole process.

We'd been back to the Hospital intermittently during the past couple of weeks as they needed to check on my well-being and to check that I was still managing my injections without any problems.

The 14th February 1990 was the date I was to start my second set of injections, these would stimulate my follicles, therefore producing lots of lovely eggs that could be fertilised. I would administer this injection in my stomach which somehow seemed a lot less barbaric due to the amount of squidgy fat in that area. The nurse brought my medication into the treatment room and began to talk me through it, but all I could focus on was the size of that needle. It was huge. This had to be a joke, was it April fools day or something? How on earth was I going to inject myself with that? I mean if I put that in my stomach it would exit my back. It was at least double the size of the previous needle. Again I felt desperately afraid, scared, well petrified to be honest, but Lloyd quickly pointed out to me how I'd felt before the first set of injections, he also reminded me how easy I'd found them, he even offered to help me! I think that's what clinched it. The thought of a man with the use of only one arm, brandishing a needle that size in my direction didn't bear thinking about so I took the syringe, gritted my teeth, put a smile or maybe a grimace on my face and I just went for it. I carefully inserted the needle. Once positioned, I carried out my checks as I'd been shown and then slowly very slowly plunged the liquid in. I remember a strange sensation as the liquid dispersed and as I removed the syringe I remember gently rubbing my stomach in slow circular movements which felt soothing. The nurse explained that this was a good practice to adopt as it helped to distribute the medicine evenly. Once again I felt like a genius and once again it was a lot easier than I'd expected.

We left the hospital armed with our freezer bag full of drugs and headed for home. Lloyd made me feel 10 feet tall as he gushed about my bravery. There was something extremely satisfying about having the person you idolised in awe of your own capabilities, it was like role reversal and I don't know to this day, whether he did this to drive me on and give me the ability to 'keep on keeping on', or whether he truly was impressed with my courage. One day I'd pursue the answer but for now I was more than happy just to be his heroine. It was the first time in my whole life that I'd felt this way, yes I actually felt like the leader.

I carried on with these daily injections like a true professional returning to St Mary's on the 21st

February for a vaginal ultrasound and blood tests. The ultrasound monitors the growth of each follicle and the blood tests check for signs of hyper-stimulation amongst other things. I was quietly worried about the vaginal ultrasound as I imagined it would be very painful not to mention cringingly embarrassing. We arrived early at the hospital and waited somewhat nervously in the waiting room. I was called in for my blood test first. This didn't phase me at all. Then it was back to the waiting room to sweat it out until they called me for my ultrasound. Lloyd asked if I'd rather go in on my own, bless him, always the gent, not wanting to add to what we already perceived to be a very embarrassing situation, but I actually wanted him there to hold my hand. The nurse showed me the probe, which for all intense and purposes looked somewhat like a vibrator and I remember thinking 'maybe this wouldn't be so bad after all!' The radiographer then placed a sheath over the probe and applied lots of warm lubricant and as she began to insert it, I prayed 'please Lord don't let me trump now!' Suffice to say it wasn't anything like I'd first imagined and the whole process was very informative as she talked us through everything she was doing and explained everything she was seeing on the screen pointing out all the follicles and confirming to us that my body was responding exactly how it should. YIPPEE another stage under out belts, this really was a piece of cake.

Following my scan we went back to the waiting room for yet another wait to see the nurse. It wasn't long before we were shown into the office and advised to carry on with the injections but we'd need to come back in 4 days for another ultrasound and blood test. They were very thorough and we were both impressed with how well we were treated throughout the whole process by everyone we met. As we left the Hospital that day I remember commenting that the doctors and nurses that chose to help infertile couples must be hand-picked for their utter kindness and their ability to empathise the situation. I wondered how many of them were childless, not that it mattered one iota but I would have loved to have known.

By Tuesday the 27th February I was in full bloom. My ovaries were ready. I had produced a full crop and I felt extremely proud, I would have strutted around with my puffed out chest only by this stage my stomach was somewhat sore and I was looking forward to offloading my crop as soon as possible. We were instructed to return to the Hospital at 11pm that evening for an injection which had to be administered by a nurse and this injection would help the release of the eggs the following day when I was to return and have my crop harvested by way of ultrasound for which I would be anaesthetised, and I love being anaesthetised.

I was up bright and early the following morning and I hadn't had a bite to eat since 10pm the night before, as instructed, due to the fact that I was to undergo my minor op for the harvesting of my lovely eggs. I have to stress that the journey the night before had been an absolute nightmare due to the number of takeaways and restaurants we'd passed. The fact that I had only just eaten mattered not a jot because I knew that I couldn't even have a cup of tea from then until after my op the next day and therefore I wanted to eat and drink everything in sight and boy it all smelt delicious! Funny the things we notice when we're faced with any kind of abstinence.

I was over the moon that they'd managed to collect 22 eggs, how good am I? Now it would be the turn of Lloyd's 5 star sperm to carry out their duty and I had no doubt in my mind that we were well on the way to our first baby and I left the hospital that day with a spring in my step and a huge smile on my face. Nothing could get me down, I felt as light as a feather and it had nothing to do with the fact that my poor swollen ovaries had been relieved from their heavy burden of 11 follicles each.

We were both ecstatic to learn that all 22 eggs had fertilised. Six numbers on a Saturday night couldn't even come close to the exhilaration we both felt. We were hugging and kissing and dancing and making merry, neither of us could sit still. We rang everyone to brag about our booty and we couldn't wait to be impregnated.

Our three embryos were replaced on Saturday the 3rd March 1990. The remaining embryos were to be frozen. It felt strange walking away and leaving 19 embryos behind, I felt as though I was being a bad parent leaving them to fend for themselves. I almost couldn't bear the thought that they would be put into a freezer. I put some of my feelings and mixed emotions down to my raging hormones and as I climbed into the car I remembered that the doctor had suggested I go home, relax and have lots of happy thoughts. We were to return to the hospital on Friday 16th March for the blood test that would prove our pregnant state. I was going to stay positive, I would be happy; I wanted to give my embryos the best chance I could.

That fortnight was the longest in history and there was no way I could take my mind off my embryos. I became afraid to go to the toilet for fear the embryos might fall out, so as ridiculous as it sounds I would take Lloyd with me for support. He never complained and he never belittled my fears though he must have thought me a crackpot.

We tried to fill this fortnight with fun. We'd go on walks or we'd watch our favourite films, we almost wore out Frank Capra's 'It's A Wonderful Life'. A beautiful story about a man called George Bailey, played by James Stewart, filmed around the Christmas period. George becomes disenchanted with life's cruel challenges and concludes that his family and friends would be better off without him. It's at this point George receives life's greatest gift! It has a powerful message and would warm the heart of anyone. We so love this film and I found out many years later that it was also one of my Grandmother's favourite films too.

Fortunately the hours passed and so did the days and when Friday arrived we attended St Mary's. They were very considerate, there was no waiting whatsoever. We entered the hospital and undertook the blood test immediately. We found ourselves in the canteen having a cup of tea while we awaited our fate.

We ambled back to the office at a snails pace due to the apprehension we both felt as we were fully aware this result would change our lives forever no matter what the outcome. This was probably the hardest part of all. I was desperate to feel upbeat and positive but because the rest of our lives hinged on this moment, the pressure was almost unbearable. I remember the hollow sound of our shoes on the hard floor and I remember thinking that I wanted the corridor to be at least another mile long to enable me to hold onto my dream a while longer. I had an immense feeling of impending doom and I could tell Lloyd was uneasy too. We tried to be flip and light-hearted in order to encourage each other, we've always done this but it didn't come easy this time for either of us.

"Whatever happens remember to stay strong", Lloyd proffered. "Stay strong and positive if it's failed sweetie in order to heal quickly and get back in the zone. But stay strong if we've succeeded to give our baby the best chance at survival". I smiled at him and thought to myself 'there is no baby' I could just sense it. I could already feel the ache in my chest. My breathing was staggered and I could feel my chin quiver. I was fighting away the dreaded despair welling up inside of me I was desperate to feel positive. I therefore attempted to revisit the feelings I had earlier in the month as I'd injected myself and became Lloyd's hero. But it was no use because this old hero was about to fall and about to fall hard.

Lloyd's 30th Birthday was next Tuesday and I'd had every intention of throwing him a birthday bash fit for a king, but something stopped me. Instead I'd chosen to take him to the Theatre, Les Miserables was playing at the Palace in Manchester and so I booked a box to mark the occasion. I would take him to dinner and then surprise him with the production. I guess with hindsight I'd chosen to celebrate his birthday this way to accommodate a failure, therefore avoiding the 'tea and sympathy' that we would have had to endure from all our kind-hearted friends had I thrown a party.

Subconsciously I pictured our success and thought that the evening belonged to just the two of us. We could celebrate our pregnancy with family and friends at a later date. Either way we were to spend the evening on our own as I knew this was for the best.

"Trudie and Lloyd Thompson please", our names were called. We glanced at each other, took deep breaths and followed the nurse into the treatment room. 'Oh! Please please please don't say it', I was desperately thinking while in anguish grinding my teeth. If she delivered a negative result now I saw myself just collapsing in a heap.

She waited until we were seated, "I am so very sorry..............." and there it was. The words were out. My mouth was dry, my heart was thumping, and my despair was clearly visible as my face contorted. I couldn't hear a word even though all my senses seemed heightened and I gulped in air as I began to shake with the shock. My eyes were wide open almost cartoon like as I tried to stop my tears flowing. I was alone, so horribly alone, I couldn't breathe, this wasn't fair, I was a good person, I deserved to be happy, I needed my baby, I loved my baby, I couldn't live like this. Why oh why was this my fate? No one could have understood the depression I was spiralling into. I sat numb staring at the wall as I tried to overcome my sense of inadequacy and frustration. I wanted to pull my hair out and scream at the heavens - I wanted to demand to know why I wasn't pregnant. Why didn't my body function the way other women's bodies did? I asked myself these question over and over, time and time again but even the experts couldn't explain.

Eventually I would have my baby I had to believe that. But it was taking so much longer than I'd ever imagined. The waiting was the most maddening. I had to wait for the medical appointments. I had to wait for the tests, wait for the treatments and wait and wait and wait. I had no privacy or modesty. I hated it. I was fed up centring my world around my menstrual cycle, which constantly played mind games with me. My period would turn up a day late or two days late and it broke my heart every time. But this time I knew my period would turn up because I'd just been told and I was wallowing around in my self pity. I was running out of time, my biological clock was ticking away faster and faster I needed to get straight

Dreams Do Come True

back on it. I needed to get this period out of the way so I could have some of my frozen embryos replaced.

I was losing my mind but no one was noticing, not even Lloyd. We rose from our seats, said our goodbyes and left the surgery. I was very grateful for the long walk to the car park which we undertook in complete silence neither one of us wanting to say the wrong thing. Neither one of us knowing what to say. How could you take away the pain, how could you make it better?

I know that everyone thought me obsessive and moody but I was living my life in fear. I was afraid so terribly afraid.

Our love making had for many years now taken on a very routine quality as we would still try to conceive naturally. Lloyd hated sex on a schedule probably as much as I did but it was a case of 'needs must' though I was also afraid that at some stage this might break us… That was why it was so important that the IVF had to work, it just had to because I wanted to keep my marriage, correction I was desperate to keep my marriage, but yet again my body had failed me, it had failed us!

I was willing to do anything. I was willing to do everything. I would sacrifice all in my quest to fulfil my longing. I'd already given up cigarettes, alcohol, fatty foods and caffeine. I avoided so many foods.

My life truly was on hold, I'd given up on a major career choosing to put my desire for a family first.

On the journey home I practised sheer determination in an effort to put my mind in a place where it would be able to heal my body and more importantly, my soul. I pictured myself making the numerous phone calls to family and friends as quickly as possible delivering the news as I knew they would be on tenterhooks waiting. But I wondered how on earth I would be strong enough to convince them that the diagnosis meant we were closer to our goal. I didn't want their sympathy as sympathy would only impact on the 'woe is me' attitude I didn't want to sink into. And I certainly didn't want people to be afraid of me. I didn't want my dear family walking on eggshells not knowing how to behave around me. I wanted to be strong for them as much as anything. I'd put my best foot forward like I always did, I searched down in my soul and I knew my prayers would be answered one day, just not today.

I was aware that Lloyd didn't want to broach the subject of his birthday so I took the leap for him, "You've still got something to look forward to". There I'd spoken. "I think you'll enjoy your birthday treat".

"You haven't spent too much have you sweetie? After all it's just another day, just another birthday" Lloyd replied. "You'll have to wait and see", I smiled.

I was strong again; I'd pulled myself through and in quick-smart time. I'll put on a show that even Lloyd will be proud of. I wasn't going to let this blip destroy his day. Oh this was supposed to be so very different, I was supposed to be pregnant, that was going to be my present to Lloyd but all I had now was a meal out and the theatre and somehow it just didn't seem enough. Poor Lloyd, I was so sorry that he was saddled with a barren spouse. One day, just one day my birthday present to Lloyd would be a baby I knew in my heart of hearts that that was how it would all pan out but for now I needed to shelve my pain, yes my pain could wait for another day but for now I would continue with my plans to make Lloyd's 30th a memorable day.

I'd booked the theatre for the Saturday evening. On Saturday morning I took Lloyd breakfast in bed where I gave him his cards and presents and a cake with a candle and I even managed to sing (very badly) happy birthday. It's important to make people feel special on their day. I could see his gratitude for my efforts, it was an unspoken respect we had. I ran him a bubble bath and we got ready for our evening out very slowly and leisurely. I surprised myself how well I was handling my emotions I'd managed to put myself on the back burner for my lovely husband and I was utterly determined that we would find fun in this lovely sunny day.

So we headed out for Manchester and for once we weren't hospital bound. Funny how I'd become familiar with this vast city due to my infertility. Some things in life are quite bizarre. We ate in China Town and for once I didn't pay any attention to the ingredients I just ate everything I wanted and I had pudding too. I also consumed alcohol and was quite tipsy after just one glass of wine. It felt good. We talked while we ate about all manner of subjects we even touched on the failure of the previous day. Though we didn't dwell. I was so glad it was just the two of us and I hoped that Lloyd was relieved too. Just the two of us stepping out and learning how to heal with dignity.

The meal over we walked arms linked, to the theatre. We were shown to our box and very impressive it was too. It would seat up to six people and we had it all to ourselves, how privileged were we? And how extravagant was this? Lloyd was impressed! I was so pleased not to mention relieved and as the theatre lights gradually dimmed we took our seats and I for one was looking forward to getting completely caught up and lost in the drama of this most wonderful production. I'd read all the reviews and I couldn't wait to see what all the fuss was about.

Les Miserables begins in 1815 and is the story of Jean Valjean who was imprisoned for 19 years hard labour for breaking a window and stealing bread for his sister's sick child. On release the yellow card he is required to carry by law identifies him as a former prisoner! This obviously creates many problems for him. He is befriended by The Bishop of Digne but the desperate Valjean repays The Bishop by stealing a silver plate. He is soon caught by the Police but the kind Bishop supports Valjean and confirms that he had given Valjean the silver - it is at this point Valjean decides to forget his past and start a new life. He works very hard and eventually became the owner of a factory in northern France, he changed his name and he also became the town's Mayor.

This is the tale of a man's struggle to live through injustice and revolution, his life spans from chain gang, to outcast and fugitive but he died a hero.

There is love, compassion and deceit in this magnificent production and it carried me away, just as I'd known it would do. There was also the added bonus that it was appropriate to cry which I did. I cried a bucket-load of tears and I do believe Lloyd shed a tear or two. We cried for the injustice that Valjean had had to endure through his life. We cried for the effort he put into being a good person, an unselfish, kind and loving man who cared so much for the people around him. But in truth we cried more for the injustice that we felt. The hand we'd been dealt and the road we were travelling that was far too cruel.

We eventually left the theatre later that night having started the inevitable healing process. The production itself had given us drive, we both felt lifted and we both knew that on Monday morning we would call the Hospital and we would once again arrange to begin the journey that would eventually lead us to our dream only this time the cycle would be a lot less daunting as I could start to use my frozen embryos - yes, it truly is a wonderful life!

The Success

Trudie:

'A whole 6 weeks', I thought grumpily before the next scan, how the hell was I gonna survive a whole 6 weeks? Well there was nothing I could do but bite the bullet and crack on with it, after all it was only time! I could read about having babies. I could knit something beautiful for my baby. I could watch DVD's about having babies and being a parent, but I knew I wouldn't do any of the above as that would be accepting all was going to be well in this pregnancy and this after all was me we were talking about, and 'all going well' just didn't happen to me. Whatever I do I mustn't get carried away with the excitement of maybe giving birth one day.

We drove home. I don't think we spoke much on that journey. As for me I kept swinging from sheer deliriousness to complete depression, not quite sure what to think or feel. I noticed that I did, every now and again, start stroking my stomach desperately hoping that Lloyd hadn't noticed. I didn't want him to think I'd lost the plot but by stroking my tummy I felt as though I was closer to my foetus, oh what a lovely word 'foetus'. I wondered what my foetus looked like as we drove from Manchester, I must take a look in one of my many pregnancy books when I get home. Or maybe not, wouldn't some say that that could be construed as 'counting one's chickens'? But I really wanted to see what a foetus looked like at 6 weeks. Would it have arms and legs yet?

Who knows? Would it look like a baby?

"What're you thinking?" cut in Lloyd. "You look a million miles away". I was. I was on cloud nine and for me that was about as far away as one could get.

"I want to be in labour", came my reply.

"Eh? Why don't you just enjoy the pregnancy first?"

"Too scared", I couldn't even articulate how afraid I truly was. I was too scared to be sat in the car, just in case some other foolish selfish road user came too close and ended up running into us. I was too scared to stand up and walk. I was too scared to get out of the car on our arrival home in case one of the neighbours fancied a chat. I was too scared to think that maybe one day I'd give birth but most of all I was too scared not to become someone's mum!

'Afraid of your own shadow', Lloyd always used to say and I'll hold my hands up, yup that was me Mrs. Too Scared. How can you enjoy life if you're too scared? I don't know. I've been too scared for as long as I can remember and on the odd occasion when I allowed myself the pleasures of not being afraid I'd have a wonderful time but then Too Scared takes over again. Maybe I'm just cautious as I like to dot my i's and cross my t's, not take risks. I like to cover all eventualities so that nothing shocks me. But at this moment in my life I needed to be positive and I needed to have happy thoughts because that's what those lovely, wonderful, kind, special, hand-picked IVF doctors and nurses always say. So I must adopt the Great British pass-time and get myself one of those stiff upper lips. I must allow myself the thrill of emotions that pregnancy brings and I shall be one of the happiest people alive and lets face it I had everything to be happy about.

We pulled up at home, home sweet home, I now truly understood that saying. I love my home and I didn't care that it was practically falling down. It was beautiful and one day I would do it justice. This will be a happy home for our child to grow up in, it already had a bucket load of memories some sad but boy the good were exceptional! I glanced around, the coast was clear so I moved as swiftly as my pregnant state would allow, phew, I was through the gate and Lloyd was close behind me, he overtook me and put the key in the door I almost grappled him to the floor once the door was opened in my haste to enter. Once inside I pulled Lloyd though the doorway and slammed it shut! Hurray, we'd made it. We'd survived our journey and I was never ever going to leave until I went into the labour. I was gonna cocoon myself away. I ran to get my books and quickly flicked through the pages looking for a picture of my foetus. Back and forth I went, less haste more speed, I thought. There it was, a foetus, but this foetus was 8 weeks which was 2 weeks ahead of me. I searched and searched but couldn't find a 6 week old foetus so I decided I'd just make the 8 week one a wee bit smaller. That should do. So there it was my very own little kidney bean. I have never been more proud of my performance in my life.

I had to find Lloyd and show him what our kidney bean looked like. Now where'd he gone? I soon found him in the kitchen making bacon butties and brews. I thrust the book in his face and pointed. He glanced but didn't really know what I was showing him. "Our baby!" I cried, "That's what our baby looks like! Well a little smaller but none the less... That is what he/she looks like". And with that I puffed my chest out, how clever were we?

I picked up the phone and rang mum immediately as I wanted to update her with all the news. Poor mum was like poor Lloyd. They'd both been dragged through this IVF experience and her nerves were probably just as jaded as Lloyd's but she hid it better, years of experience you see. And as the phone rang my mind drifted back to a time when I wasn't going to be able to undertake my final programme, this cycle, because finances dictated that we were brassic, skint, poor, broke. There was no money left for IVF, or anything else for that matter, then in came my lovely parents, "You must take this money", they had offered on hearing the news that it was all over for us. Bless them, they had been saving up for double glazing and they were offering us the savings they had diligently put by. How on earth could we take it? We'd lost all our own money. We'd re-mortgaged our house and it was one thing to lose your own money but to lose someone else's just wasn't right. Which ever way I looked at it, and trust me I looked long and hard at it, but I just couldn't justify taking it. The wind would howl through their rotten wooden windows and they weren't as young as they once were and here we were contemplating taking their hard-earned cash that they'd diligently saved. It just didn't feel right. They were, and still are the most selfless people on the planet bar none!

Lloyd convinced me that we needed to take the money as it was our only chance and he thought it was a good omen. Therefore I begrudgingly, but ever so gratefully, took their savings but I couldn't help feeling that we might just as well burn the money because it had as much chance of success as I had of actually conceiving a baby or winning the lottery!

"Hello", mum's voice jolted me back to reality. "Oh! Mum you should see our baby he's beautiful".

I rambled on and on and as always she just listened quietly without interrupting. I talked about the scan and how he looked like a kidney bean in my books. For some reason I had started to always refer to him as 'he', maybe it was a sixth sense, I really don't know, but I had noticed this. I talked to mum for hours telling her my fears and she was always comforting and very calming.

Lloyd presented me with my bacon sarni and cup of tea, it was yummy. Was I allowed bacon butties in my state? I had a lot of research to do, I knew about the obvious rules but I'd never read anywhere that you couldn't eat bacon! Mum put my mind at rest and I tucked in.

The days, weeks and eventually the months passed and I grew to immense proportions, I was truly becoming obese, I was absolutely huge and it was very hard to get about. My stomach was rock hard and very uncomfortable. I was so big that I couldn't get up if I was resting on my back, something you're not supposed to do at the end of pregnancy. But I would flail my arms and legs around in my desperate attempt to attain some leverage, then once on my side I'd push myself up on my arms, swinging my legs underneath me and I don't mind admitting it used to thoroughly wear me out.

I did try to keep fit and active. I would walk to my parents' house for lunch. It was about 2 miles but I'd take my time and it was always pleasant. On one such walk I ended up with cramps in my side, maybe I was walking too fast and it was just stitch, or maybe the baby was uncomfortable but whatever it was it was excruciatingly painful. I persevered as I was only a few hundred yards away from a bench so I could have a sit and catch my breath once I reached it.

It seemed an awful long way to reach my goal but I was relieved when I did and I plonked my weary bones down and took some big gulps of air whilst rubbing my pain. I must have looked quite a distressed sight because not before too long a white van pulled up and a workman jumped out and raced towards me thrusting a mobile phone in my direction whilst all the time encouraging me to take deep breaths and stay calm! He didn't look calm! Then it hit me, poor bloke thought I was giving birth! Bless him I'm not sure many people would have stopped to assist but I assured him I was okay and I didn't have far to go and that I was just catching my breath. To this very day I am so touched by his eagerness to help, I never knew who he was but I thought he must be a very courageous young man and whenever anyone acts in such a good natured way it always makes me very proud of the human race, there are some amazing people out there in this big wide world, some lovely folk who don't mind putting themselves out and helping complete strangers.

I heaved my heavy frame off the bench and headed towards my parent's house my pain being very noticeable and I began to wonder myself if this was it.

Mum had made some of her lovely vegetable soup with lentils and we had hunks of buttered bread it was delicious, she's a very good cook and she always made plenty. As we ate we chatted about my experience.

The Birth

Trudie

I didn't want to appear rude but I wanted Lloyd to go out as there's only so much fussing one person can take… Especially one who'd grown to be as tetchy as me!

As previously mentioned, I was huge; I was so enormous you'd have needed a diversion sign in order to circumnavigate me should you have been unfortunate enough to have crossed my path had I dared to venture out!

Oh boy I couldn't wait to give birth now. This was so uncomfortable but I didn't want to moan as I was very grateful for my pregnant state. I just wanted it over now. I had spent the last 12 years moaning about not having a pregnancy and now I wanted to whinge about actually having a pregnancy - there really is no pleasing some folk!

I know I was becoming painful to live with or be around I would love to know how the heck women did this more than once or why they actually wanted to do this more than once? I couldn't move, I couldn't breathe, I couldn't eat and I most certainly couldn't sleep. Bedtime was dreadful because this was the time my cherub decided he wanted desperately to play. During the daylight hours he would be rocked and lulled with my movement, my voice or the sound of the TV or radio so he would sleep and sleep then at night he would come alive and practice his tap-dancing routine or his sit ups or sometimes he would use my ribcage in order to carry out a set or two of pull ups. If I lay on my side and his feet were by the mattress he would either kick or thump so hard that the mattress would vibrate and poor (uncomplaining) Lloyd would be shaken awake. If I cuddled up to Lloyd and my sweet cherub could feel Daddies back he would kick him, again jolting him out of any sleep he may have been having. It was decided I should sleep in another room so that Lloyd could rest.

I was bruised and battered but didn't want to say anything to anyone for fear of sounding ungrateful.

I was three weeks away from my due date and Lloyd was invited on a friend's stag night in Southport. He was unsure about leaving me but I was more than happy for him to go. I wanted him to go out, let his hair down, have a few drinks do whatever it was that lads do on stag nights. He eventually agreed and took his mobile phone with him just in case!

After he'd left I made a phone call to an old friend who was also pregnant, with her third! As we chatted I began to feel really unwell and tired so I cut the conversation short, made a cup of hot chocolate and went upstairs to bed to have a read. I think I only managed to read a page or so as my eyes were drooping so I made the most of the fact that I could feel no wriggling in my tummy therefore a good indication that 'baby boy' was snoozing so I snuggled down to catch some shut eye even though it was only 9 o'clock. I went out like a light. Two hours later though I was awoken by a thump in my stomach which made me shoot bolt upright. I wasn't in pain, but not only did I feel the thump I could have sworn I heard it too. Then I felt wet! Oh lordy I was peeing the bed I jumped out and ran to the loo. I just couldn't stop. I looked down and there was blood, not a lot, just a smattering. Then it dawned on me, my waters had broken. I rolled up a towel, shoved it between my legs and waddled back to the bedroom to ring the hospital and ask their advice. What would happen next? How much time did I have? Why wasn't I in excruciating pain like they show on TV? Did I have time for a bath? The questions went on and on some making sense some not but my mind rambled away on its own planet quite happily.

I dialled the number I'd been given and for once in my life I was so glad that I was organized. I knew where everything was and I was more than prepared. I was obviously hoping the doctors and nurses would give top-marks for my efforts and maybe even hold me up as a shining example for all to take notes in how to conduct oneself! Rambling on you see… The nurse answered the phone bringing me back to reality. After I'd explained the situation she asked me to get to the hospital explaining that my baby was no longer in a sterile environment.

By now it was 11.30pm on Saturday 27th February 1999, and the nurse had made me promise not to drive myself. Personally I didn't know what all the fuss was about. It was late and I didn't want to pester anyone. Then I remembered… maybe I should contact Lloyd. I rang his mobile. On answering he bellowed down the phone, "Hold on, I'm going outside, bit noisy in here… hic…" He babbled on slurring slightly whilst, I assumed, walking out of the nightclub. He chatted to a few people en route as he made his way to take his call. He had a bit of banter with the doormen, I just assumed he knew them but apparently he'd been boring everyone with his imminent fatherhood situation.

At last there was peace and quiet. "Allo", he was usually so eloquent when speaking on the phone but tonight you could tell he'd been out and was more than a touch squiffy. It crossed my mind just to enquire as to his evening and bid him goodnight but this was at the point of my very first contraction which took me by surprise, though with hindsight I guess it was nature's way of saying "Tell him".

"Hiya, sweetie hope you're having a good time..." I started but he cut in "I'm having a ball, feel a bit bad on Mel coz, even though I'm trying, I feel like I'm hogging all the limelight but I just can't shut up, don't know whether it's the drink or what, but I can't shut up! We've had every conceivable shot there is. We've been in all the trendy bars some I've never been in before and some you just wouldn't recognise. I mean when was the last time we had a night out in Southport? I've gotta bring you, you'll love it, very Parisian..."

I did eventually manage to get a word in, which was very unusual because Lloyd has never been the verbal diarrhoea type, he's more the 'listen to everyone, get all the information then come out with a one-line corker to knock em all dead type!'

"He's on his way," was all I remember saying which was met with complete silence. "My waters have broken and he's on his way" I repeated. I was just so excited my heart was thumping and it was so good to say those words, it's a moment I'll always remember and absolutely treasure. I remember the green wallpaper; I remember the awful wardrobes that were painted the same colour as the wallpaper. I remember the ready-made cheap tacky curtains I'd hung up ages ago thinking that they'll do until we needed the room for something. But most of all I remember thinking 'when I come home I'll be a mum'!

Lloyd coughed and spluttered his way through a few sentences about the fact that he'd already arranged a lift 'just in case'. And he'd be with me as soon as he could. I could hear him sobering up and I remember thinking, what a shame as he hadn't had a good night out in such a long time and he was having such a great evening. I assured him that he had plenty of time as I hadn't even had my second contraction yet and I was only going to the Hospital as I'd been summoned by the nurse, who was probably just covering her own backside.

Although I didn't want to, due to the lateness of the hour, I rang mum and asked if she could give me a lift to the Hospital. Like she'd say 'no'! She always helped. She will help anyone and she never ever complained about how hard she worked or how much her family drained her. She is always so happy to help, so I knew she wouldn't mind but I hated to bother her.

Suffice to say she got to me here quick smart. "You must have broken some speed limits", but she assured me she hadn't. We had a pleasant uneventful trip to Preston. Mum dropped me at the door of the maternity unit and went to park the car plus she insisted on carrying my bag.

Once inside I was taken to the delivery suite so they could monitor my progress. How disappointing, I was only 1cm dilated. Flippin' heck this was gonna take some time and I was so desperate to meet this wee chap. I lay back on the bed, mum was telling me not to be too disappointed and at least I was in labour, my waters had actually broken I hadn't just wet myself. And they were letting me stay, not sending me packing. I felt sick, and then I vomited. The nurse explained that this was quite natural as it was the surge of hormones. I really didn't feel well at all, I was too hot, I kept throwing up then I had diarrhoea. This wasn't how it was supposed to be, I was supposed to be elegant and ladylike not trumping and puking.

Mum was very soothing and as always very kind she would place cool hands or a cool cloth on my head. The pains were starting to come thick and fast so the chances of having a doze and sleeping my way through to the birth stage were completely out of the question. All the time the doctors and nurses would pop in and check on me. I remember working out that my pains were lasting for the count of 15 so when I could feel one on the way I would start counting one and two and three and four and... All the time focusing on a pretty flower I'd spotted on the wallpaper... and ten... At which point I knew it would soon be over for a minute or so until the next one.

Once I'd found this method helped I felt quite calm, each pain would bring with it the excitement of meeting the most important person that would ever come into my life. The person for whom my whole life had been about. The whole purpose of me.

For some reason the music to the Rocky films kept going through my head. I felt as though by giving birth I was about to save the world.

The door flew open with such ferocity it practically came off its hinges! And there he stood the man of my dreams, swaying. He stumbled towards me, was he going to fall on me, was he crying? He smelt horrendous, a concoction of strong alcohol and smoke. Bless him he must have tried to sober up on the way back I'd completely forgotten... one and two and three and. And fifteen. I smiled up at him and turned to explain to the doctors that he didn't really drink and he never smoked and that he was on a night out for a friend's stag party. Well, I didn't want them informing Social Services.

Lloyd was very Del Boy in his approached which I put down to the amount of alcohol he must have consumed, and I can recall him asking the doctors which end they needed him! Poor Lloyd he was trying so hard to sober up and just be Lloyd. You could see his desperate desire to be the sober Lloyd. The Lloyd who knew how to behave in any situation.

The Lloyd who was good at making decision. The Lloyd who was always professional in his conduct.

He kissed and cuddled me lots... one and two and three and four and... He told me how proud he was of me. He told me how ladylike and refined I was and that I had always been his heroine but that I was 50 times more his heroine tonight and he felt as though he was going to explode with the amount of love and pride he had caged up inside him. His ramblings were most definitely alcohol induced though I do believe he meant every word he said. He kept asking if there was anything he could do to help.

Eventually one of the doctors suggested that maybe he should sit with mum. He swung round, "I had no idea you were here", he slurred at her, "when did your mum come?" he turned to me, "she brought me"... one and two and three and four..."and she's gonna take you home for a sleep and sober up".

The doctors agreed that Lloyd should go and get some rest and come back in the morning so mum and Lloyd left.

The pain was wearing me down so I'd taken to the gas and air and the medical team asked if I would like an epidural, not something I'd planned but maybe I should, so I agreed to have a mini-epidural. The epidural was administered and by now there were more medics arriving and I knew deep down that all was not well!

All through the night I was monitored. More and more staff appeared. At some point I must have dozed off but I didn't get much sleep as my mini epidural numbed the pain but it didn't eradicate it altogether. I must have slept through some of my contractions with pure exhaustion but it was a long very uncomfortable night. I remember having a walk around trying to speed the process up.

I was so glad to see Lloyd when he returned in the morning. He was all spruced up and looking delicious. He made enquiries as to my well-being and asked the staff how things were going. No one gave anything away but I was aware all was not well, there were far too many people checking me. I just had a feeling!

One of the nurses asked that in between my next contraction I get into a wheelchair as they wanted to take me for a scan. I tried to stay calm. I'm no medic but surely this isn't the norm. I was also aware that Lloyd was watching my every move; maybe even he was aware that things weren't how you'd say tickety-boo!

I could feel my next pain building so as instructed I heaved my huge bulk into the waiting wheelchair and immediately grabbed for the gas and air to alleviate the tension I was feeling. The pain I could deal with, it was the fear of not giving birth that was causing me the most stress. I kept smiling for the sake of my lovely husband. We motored at such speed down those corridors, Jeremy Clarkson would have been astounded, I'm quite sure we rounded 'Gambon' twice - this again increased my worry. We flew through the doors of the x-ray department;

luckily I was just about managing to keep my dignity. We were met with a sea of faces and I remember being alarmed at how many people were in the waiting room on a Sunday. They all seemed to be staring in my direction but then again I must have cut a ridiculous sight, they probably believed me to be a practical joke - so where's Beadle? And was I laughing? I was huffing and puffing and I swear I could have blown any house down, wolf-style. I was sweating and grinding my teeth into my mouth piece. My hair was stuck to my head and there wasn't a scrap of make-up to be seen. I must have been in pain because I'm the type who won't bring the milk in without my eyebrows and a smidge of lippy.

We had obviously queue jumped due to my predicament and I was dutifully whizzed straight in. The radiographer was waiting and it was quite obvious she'd been fully briefed. She was calm. She was the only person who was calm. She asked me to jump onto the bed she was patting gently with her hand. I could no sooner have jumped than I could have run the London marathon! Stupid woman I thought, do I look in any fit state to jump? Again not wanting to distress Lloyd, I waited for my moment… And ten… And eleven… And twelve… And thirteen… I could just about make it so I took my chance. Thankfully I surprised myself with my athleticism, I didn't let go of my gas and air, I'd come to the decision that this was my lifeline and I wasn't gonna give it up in a hurry.

The calm but stupid radiographer was suggesting I lay down flat to enable her to gain access to my abdominal region! Someone give me a gun, she's had it! She has obviously never ever EVER given birth; my pain was such that I couldn't have straightened my body if my life had depended on it. So I just sat there, knees raised, arms behind me supporting my weight and this was the best I could muster so it was this position or nothing she'd just have to do her best.

She obviously realised that I was a woman very close to the edge by now so she gave it her best shot. At least she'd warmed the jelly.

Within minutes I was being jet propelled back along the corridors only this time we were heading towards the theatre. I was being asked to sign consent forms en route. There were doctors, nurses, porters then there was Lloyd. He looked ashen, drained and so worried. The noise was immense, there were orders being barked out, doors where swinging back and forth with the comings and goings of the hospital personnel. I remember thinking just cut me open and get my baby out alive, stop faffing. As they wheeled me through the theatre door I could see Lloyd hovering, not really knowing what was going on and not really knowing what he should do to appease this awful nightmarish situation we now found ourselves in. I remember smiling at him and mouthing the words, "I'm so sorry", and I gave him the thumbs up then blackness.

I don't know whether you've ever been put to sleep for an operation or procedure but as far as I'm concerned it's one of the best experiences ever, absolutely brilliant. I'd become addicted over the years, in fact whenever I was informed of an impending operation, secretly I was overjoyed because I loved the sensation of being put to sleep. I'd play a game with myself and try to stay awake for as long as possible. After I could feel the gas creeping up my arm, across my shoulder and up into my head, just then, as I could smell the gas, I'd fall under! Great! The government should provide a bedtime service every night for every household. The NHS should visit every home in Britain and offer a 'put to sleep injection'. No more insomniacs and no more tired folk. Brilliant! Stroke of genius! We'd have a pleasant, well rested, smiling nation.

"Trudie", I could hear my name. It was being spoken very softly, I liked it and therefore I snoozed on.

"Trudie", Again there was that angelic voice.

"Trudie", I managed to squint. Someone was standing over me. I was very comfy so I carried on snoozing.

Eventually! Bam! Realisation hit. I opened my eyes and tried to move. I heard a baby cry. My vision was coming and going. I heard Lloyd's voice, it was weak, I'd never heard it that faint before. I struggled to gain consciousness, this was hopeless. Again, the cry. Did I have a baby? Was that my baby? Why can't I see? I knew my eyes were open. Maybe this would be the draw-back with putting a nation to sleep.

Then I focused. Lloyd was holding a pink bundle over me. He was crying, I mean really crying... I reached my hand up to touch my baby's face; she was beautiful, so tiny. I remember Lloyd's words, "Meet your mum".

I was asleep. It was the best sleep I think I'd ever experienced. It was a carefree sleep, for the first time I was having a carefree sleep. I don't know how long I slept for and I don't remember any sequence of events. I remember waking up with my beautiful baby in a plastic cot next to my bed, I wanted to hold her, but it was difficult to move as I was sporting a drip. A blood transfusion. There was also something attached to my leg. A catheter.

I eventually swung my legs over the edge of the bed and I positioned my drip, I shakily stood up and I remember asking if I could hold her. But there was no one there to help me. I was weak and I was glad I hadn't just tried to pick her up on my own. I was desperate to sniff her. I was desperate to kiss her and tell her how I felt.

I stood looking down at my pink bundle. I couldn't believe my luck. I could see the perfect structure to her little face. The tiny shell like ears that were so minute but oh so perfect in detail. Someone had wrapped her so tightly it looked quite cruel. There was no room for movement. It was quiet so I could hear her breathe. I didn't want to move from this moment ever. This was my moment. I was going to drink in every detail, like on my wedding day I remembered the smell of the Church as I walked down the aisle and now when I smell that smell it reminds me of the expression on Lloyd's face as our eyes met. I remember the shape of the glasses we drank champagne out of in the back of the car and I have looked everywhere for some glasses just like those. There are moments we should drink in and keep forever like a treasure locked away so that when times are hard we can recall them and they will always pull us through. This was one of those moments. There would never be a moment like this. My life's ambition was lying sleeping alive and well. I wished I could hold her but I knew I wasn't strong enough to scoop her up. I was too weak to bend over to give her a kiss and I was so tired. I managed to sit back down on my bed. I sat and I watched.

I watched my baby sleeping and I wondered how you become a good parent. I didn't ever want to let my baby down. I wanted to make nothing but good decisions, the right decisions and I wanted the decisions to come easily.

I could smell the hospital food, it smelt good. I could hear the trolley's being wheeled. I had no idea what time it was in Trudie world but I did feel hungry. Never mind the time; I had no idea what day it was on Trudie planet. I sat alone listening to the sounds and looking at my tiny miracle and wondering just what life would be like now.

Being Stags

Lloyd:

"Honestly I will be fine on my own, you go and have a good time with your mates, you can't let them down now they're expecting you".

Trudie was doing her best to convince me that she would be OK while I went on a mates 'Stag Party' in Southport. Neither of us had been on any social engagements over the past 8 months since that incredible day we found out we were pregnant. Trudie had spent the whole time 'protecting' the life that was growing inside her and we were now just 3 weeks away from meeting the precious little being we had waited all those years for.

"But you can hardly move. What if he comes early? What if…"

"Go and have a good time. I'll be fine, you deserve a break" she cut in.

She was as feisty as ever despite looking like she may pop any moment now in the later stages of pregnancy. Trudie gave the impression of being totally relaxed at the idea of me going out for the evening and her confidence made me feel it was OK to go, so I got ready for my first night out in ages. Perhaps Trudie was right? Maybe I did deserve a night out so I left the house to go and meet the guys but not before reminding her that I had my mobile with me and it would be switched on at all times.

We were meeting at Mel's house which was just a few hundred yards from where we lived. As it turned out two or three of the wives and girlfriends were having a night in while we went out and they were all aware of Trudie's condition. I was expressing my concerns about leaving her but they all reassured me she would be fine as we were still 3 weeks away from the due date.

One of the girls 'Deborah' said if there was any reason I needed to get home in a hurry then I was to just call her and she would come and get me. This was quite reassuring so off we went to be 'Stags'!

I'm still not sure why Southport was chosen as the destination for the grooms last night of freedom? Maybe he had just decided to go up market from the usual venue of Blackpool. I had only ever been on two stag parties outside of my own and both were in Blackpool and both had been a nightmare as on each occasion I had managed to miss the transport home!

This was not really my idea of a good night out, a group of guys on a pub crawl trying to get as drunk as possible as quickly as possible and being loud and leery particularly when any females appeared on the horizon.

Mind you, any females that joined our group quickly dispersed because I was not holding my drink as well as I usually do, which was not surprising since it was so long since I had been out and, the drunker I got, the more I wanted to proclaim to the world that I was going to be a dad very soon! I bored everyone and anyone who fell into earshot, doormen, barmen, waitresses, innocent passers by. I couldn't shut up. Anyone would think this was the first baby ever to be born on planet earth.

"You're scaring off the girls, harping on about your wonderful pregnant wife you dickhead" said a couple of the guys. This didn't stop me. I just gave them a lecture about the virtues of having a good night out without the need to be pulling birds and as you would expect on a stag party this went down like a lead balloon.

We moved from pub to pub in time honoured fashion and were all pretty hammered by the time we descended the steps to a very large, very dark and extremely noisy club. This was more my scene as the music was thumping. I think the lads preferred it too as no one could hear me going on about the world's first baby that was going to be born in three weeks time.

I must have finally started to chill out and get into the swing of the night because I was really surprised yet extremely relaxed about it when I could feel my mobile vibrating in my pocket.

I was still relaxed as I vaguely made out a female voice as I answered the call. I couldn't make out who was calling me or why so I said "hold on while I go outside". Still relaxed, I gave the doormen a nod as I passed them and went out into the cool night air and relative quiet. "Sorry who's that? I said into the phone.

The words that met my enquiry will stay with me for eternity; they sobered me up in an instant and froze me to the spot. I nearly dropped my phone. "It's me, my waters have broken… he's on his way".

Outwardly I think I must have appeared pretty calm but inwardly my head was in a spin. A million thoughts passed through my mind as I took stock of the news that had just been relayed to me.

12 years, 144 months of waiting was finally coming to an end. It all seemed rather surreal. Even though every day for the past few months I had seen the lump growing in Trudie, and felt it kicking and moving about I still don't think my mind was ready to accept that it would ever be anything more than just a kicking lump and it was actually going to turn into a real baby.

Before I could speak Trudie continued... "Now don't panic, I've spoken to the hospital and called my Mum and she's on her way for me, she's taking me to hospital, I'm alright"

You could have knocked me down with a feather, the collected calm with which Trudie was speaking was immense; she even asked me if I was having a good time with the lads.

"Never mind that, I'm on my way now" I said and proceeded to explain my standby arrangement with Deborah and promised to be there as quickly as possible. No way did I want to miss the birth after waiting all these years to reach this point in our lives.

Deborah thought I was having a drunken joke at first as I explained my predicament. When it became apparent that I was deadly serious she was brilliant and having arranged where to meet me she immediately jumped in her car to come and get me. I had about half an hour to wait. 30 minutes with my thoughts. I wanted to be there at the hospital now. I thought after all the waiting we had done in our lives that when the time came I would be ready but here I was caught on the hop as our baby was putting in his appearance 3 weeks early while I was away from his Mother for the first time in months.

Ironic I thought how I had spent the last few hours proclaiming his pending arrival like some religious Zealot and my words were now coming true on the same night. I smiled to myself and thought maybe his ears were burning and he needed to get out. I had induced the labour.

I remembered the lads were still downstairs in the club. I couldn't just go without telling them my news. Although they were probably enjoying the break from my proclamations of the 'second coming' I didn't want them thinking I had been abducted by aliens so I headed back inside to let them know I would be leaving shortly and why.

The collective reaction from the guys was amazing. You would have thought I was actually giving birth myself, I was a hero. Drinks were being thrust upon me amidst all the handshakes and back slapping. Maybe they were just relieved that the baby was actually on his way and they would be spared anymore ranting from 'The prophet Lloyd' "What are you going to call him?" somebody asked. This was just after the Beckham's had produced their first child 'Brooklyn' who was named after the place in which he was conceived, "Where was he conceived? Name him after that place" came one suggestion.

"I can't give him the name of a hospital" I replied. Laughter all round. "Name him after the place you were when you found out he was coming", came another suggestion. "Southport's a crap name for a kid you tosser" retorted someone else. More laughter. "No I mean name him after this place, what's it called?"

One of the lads leaned over the bar to ask the staff where we were as we were all too drunk to notice on the way in and then came back to the group with the proposed name for my son.

I believe your name plays a big part in your life and how others see you. It is so important that you have a good name with great relevance in my view and when it transpired that to be trendy like David and Victoria Beckham I would have to name my son (The) Dungeon I decided then and there to continue to give serious thought to choosing our son's name.

I was keeping my eye on my watch as I waited for the time to go and meet Debbie. The lads were plying me with celebratory drinks and I had to remind them that we were not out on my stag do. I felt rather guilty at upstaging the groom's night but he was as chuffed as anyone and it was a great excuse to buy more drinks. My temporary sobering up at the news my son was en-route was becoming a hazy distant memory.

Finally it was time to go and I left the guys to party on into the night. My timing was just perfect as Debbie pulled up just as I reached our arranged meeting place. I couldn't thank her enough as we set off for the hospital. It was a half hour drive in which she was subjected to my excitement, expectations and worries that everything would be all right. Debs had known us for many years and understood what this moment meant so could understand how I was feeling. She seemed to get us to the hospital in no time at all and waved me off as I jumped out of the car and lurched off drunkenly in the direction of the Maternity ward.

I had walked these hospital corridors many times before but it all seemed rather different under the influence of drink and I actually took a couple of wrong turns in my rush to get to Trudie, desperately hoping that I was in time for the birth. I rounded one more corner then the room I was looking for was right there in front of me. I paused momentarily to gather my thoughts before entering, deep breath then through the doors.

I swept into the room to see Trudie lying there with a doctor and a nurse attending to her, she looked up at me and smiled and the whole scene appeared to be very much under control. Not what I was expecting at all. Where were the teams of people to deliver the baby? Where were the birthing stirrups and other medical equipment?

"Right where do you want me? What can I do?" I offered far too loudly given the situation as I moved across to Trudie to give her a kiss and a hug. I must have smelt strongly of drink and smoke as Trudie started to explain to the medical people that I don't actually smoke at all or drink often but had been out on a 'stag party'.

The doctor smiled knowingly and suggested I take a seat in the corner to which he gestured. I looked over to see Laura my mother-in-law sitting there quietly. "When did you come in?" I asked again rather too loudly. "I've been here all the time," she said smiling and moved up so I could sit beside her.

I took a seat but all too quickly for the medical staff got up again and moved towards the bed once more offering my services. I wanted to help, I was impatient and wanted to meet my son. "What's the situation? How long have we got?" I enquired.

The doctor explained that even though Trudie was indeed in labour it was highly unlikely that the baby would be born that evening. His suggestion was that I should go home and get some sleep and come back in the morning and I would not miss a thing.

I read this as 'go home you loud drunken oik and leave us in peace to do our jobs without you getting in the way'. I was not convinced and looked to Trudie for reassurance. What if I went away and missed the birth? I would never forgive myself. We had been on this long journey together every step of the way and deserved to conclude this epic adventure together with me right by her side.

Trudie assured me that she thought the doctor was right and maybe I should go home and sober up. She was just as calm as when I had spoken to her on the phone when her waters had broken. This laid back approach was not the Trudie I had previously known and all of a sudden I was seeing a new side to her.

In our relationship down the years I had always taken on the role of 'the one who never gets flustered and always sort's out the situation whatever it may be' but that night part of our relationship underwent a great transformation.

It was as if from the moment Trudie really knew she was going to be a Mother something awoke inside her. A whole part of her being that had laid dormant all these years was being released. Through all the years of fighting the long hard struggle to be a Mum maybe she had found a new quality along the way.

I was always happy to make the big decisions in our relationship. I was comfortable being the one that coped. Truth be told I liked being Trudie's strength and always wanted to be her protector but that night we turned a corner and have never looked back.

That night, Trudie began to take responsibility for her, as yet, unborn child. She started to care for her incomplete family unit and still does to this day.

A lioness in the Serengeti would not protect and look out for her family with the same dedication as I have witnessed from my wonderful 'soul mate' over these many years. If you hurt one of us she feels it a hundred times more.

Time and again she demonstrates strength and resilience way beyond what people would expect on first meeting her. If one of us is threatened in anyway shape or form she comes out fighting and God help anyone who tries to hurt her family.

I have stood back and watched with admiration as she has taken on and beaten the doctors who said IVF was not for us. As she went against the medical people who were insisting our precious son should have the potentially dangerous MMR vaccination before taking him to France to have the jabs individually. I was so impressed with the way she sent packing the National company that wanted to erect a mobile phone mast in the church tower that over looks our lovely home. She has been successful in getting our son into both our first choice Primary and Secondary schools against all the odds.

I do not believe there is a woman on this earth more dedicated to her family and the upbringing of a child. In fact I would go as far as to say that The English Dictionary definition of 'Motherhood' should simply read – Trudie Thompson.

As I write this it dawns on me that maybe Trudie does not realise this is how I see her, how I feel about her but it is totally from the heart when I say these things and I should communicate them verbally more often because she deserves to know.

The Birth
(Part Two!)

Lloyd:

Have you ever awoken the morning after a good night out and wondered through the fog of your hangover, 'Did such and such really happen'? Or was it just a dream? Of course you have. Well you can just imagine how I reacted as I slowly came to from that restless uncomfortable sleep you tend to have following a night on the booze.

Only this time I was not wondering about little things like who I met or spoke to last night or which bars we had gone to until what time. There was something far more important lurking in my subconscious but trying to battle through all the units of alcohol and reach the surface of my slowly awakening mind. What time was it? What day was it? Where was Trudie? Then BANG! It hit me like a sledgehammer as the whole of the night before came flooding back to me in Technicolor and High Definition. I was going to be a dad. Maybe I was already a dad. Shit I needed to get back to the hospital. Why did I let them talk me into leaving in the first place?

I dived out of bed and headed for the bathroom. Ten minutes later I was driving up the Motorway heading for the hospital in Preston. That's when I realised there was no way I should be driving at all as I was still drunk from the night before. I reasoned with myself that if ever there was an extenuating circumstance, then this was it. If the police stopped me I would throw myself on their mercy and they would give me an escort to the hospital, or was that just something that happened in films? Luckily it was early Sunday morning and practically no other traffic on the road as I made my way carefully. How could Trudie ever forgive me if I chose this moment to kill myself in a car accident?

Mother and widow in the same day was not the plan.

I arrived safely in the car park and set off walking to the hospital building. The cold wind of this grey February morning was not pleasant but it was blowing away the cobwebs in my mind. What would I find when I reached the ward? How would Trudie be coping? Was the doctor right and would she still be in labour? Why did I not have some breakfast before setting off? I was starving and always had a good stodgy breakfast the morning after the night before but now I had more pressing matters to attend to and quickly turned my mind to them.

This was weird, for the second time in less than 12 hours I was rushing to the bedside of my labouring wife. Maybe you got an extra go when you have waited as long as we have? However this time the tense feeling of anxiety was much more acute when not dampened down by copious amounts of alcohol as with the night before. In all honesty I was equally excited yet scared at the same time. Was Trudie OK? Would the baby be OK? What the hell happens next? How do you be a Father? Would I be any good at it? I clearly remember thinking, what will he actually look like? What will he look like as he grows older? What will his voice sound like? Daft little things like this crossed my mind but they were all relevant to me. I was going to meet this person who, as far as I knew, was not yet in this world but when he arrived he would be depending on me and his mum (wow that sounded good!) to show him the ropes. Show him what life was all about. Bring him up in other words. What a responsibility. Was I up to it? Was Trudie up to it?

Yes Trudie was up to it I was sure of that. I would simply follow her lead in the parenting role. I was good at picking things up. I would be OK, wouldn't I?

This really was déjà vu day. The scene on the ward was much the same as the night before. Trudie was still in labour but it was not very advanced. She still had an air of being completely in control of what was happening to her as she explained to me what was going on. It all seemed pretty technical to me because apparently she had been 3cm dilated the night before and not much had happened and now she was 5cm dilated and needed to be 10cm before the baby's head could emerge. She was having contractions at intervals which caused her pain but was coping with it all remarkably well.

Throughout that morning everything seemed to intensify. The contractions became closer together; I could see that the pain from the contractions was becoming greater. Trudie availed herself of the 'gas and air' tube that was hanging over the headboard of the bed. Something called an epidural was discussed and Trudie was to have it administered. Still everything seemed to be going to plan at least as far as I could ascertain from my little knowledge of what was 'supposed to happen' and all the while Trudie was coping remarkably well. I still remind her to this day that even when her labour pains where at their most intense she maintained a ladylike dignity and did not use one word of bad language or threaten to punch my lights out if ever I came near her again. Or is that something else you only see on the telly?

Suddenly the atmosphere in the room changed. There were now four or five medical people in the room as opposed to the one or two as before. The doctor explained that he wanted Trudie to have a scan. They were concerned that both her blood pressure and that of the baby's was very low and they needed to take a look. We could immediately see the concern in each others eyes as they wheeled her off to the scanning room. Surely this could not be happening to us at this stage. The medical staff were doing their very best to play it down as just routine but we both knew something was seriously amiss! I felt sick to the pit of my stomach as they prepared Trudie for the scan. I'm filling up now as I write this remembering the look on her face trying to reassure me that everything was going to be fine. That is so typical of this wonderful woman in my life. Here we were after 12 years of trying for this baby, our dream appeared to be in danger of being taken from us in the cruellest of circumstances and she was apologising for letting me down, without a thought for herself.

After having the scan which confirmed the baby was in fact alive and healthy Trudie was brought back to the ward for more monitoring. There was still a great amount of concern amongst the medical team who were talking in whispers as though they did not want us to know the full details of the situation. Not a good idea where Trudie was concerned as she demanded to know what was going on. We were to get the answer to her question almost immediately as two porters were summoned to the ward and Trudie was wheeled off to theatre quick smart with me and the medical team in hot pursuit.

The doctor explained to me as we hurried along the corridors that the baby was having difficulty being born because the umbilical cord had somehow got around his neck and as he was trying to come down the birthing channel he was being strangled! They were rushing Trudie down to theatre to have an emergency Caesarean section.

How could this be happening to us? Was 12 years of pain and heartache not enough? I wanted to get close to Trudie, to hold her hand, kiss her and reassure her, remind her that we always come through everything together and this would be no different but such was the panic to get her to theatre that I never even got close to her. The theatre doors were flung open and the whole team of people went inside, Trudie attempting to smile and giving me the thumbs up before disappearing from my view. My natural instinct of course was to follow but I was stopped abruptly in my tracks by a nurse who told me I had to wait outside. I started to protest but she was adamant that I could not go in.

I sat outside the room waiting while various hospital staff scurried about their duties, up and down the corridor and on a couple of occasions coming out of the Theatre. Each time I looked up expectantly but no one had any news for me. I don't know how long I waited there, it could have been five minutes or fifty minutes, I honestly could not tell you even now. I don't remember because by this stage my mind was numb. I don't remember a single thought I had because I was just waiting. I was not sat there in the role of expectant father I was playing the role of waiting and hoping to be father.

I heard a baby crying and looked up. The sound was coming from the direction of the doors through which Trudie had disappeared five or fifty minutes ago but did not register as being significant, after all we were in a maternity ward and crying babies would be the norm I thought to myself.

My mind must have shut down again, maybe I was tired from lack of sleep and the drama of the day but the next few minutes again drew a blank in my memory. I remember closing my eyes, I may even have said a prayer, highly unlikely because I don't do religion but the situation needed some divine intervention.

"Mr Thompson?" I opened my eyes and looked up to see who was addressing me. The nurse was standing in front of me cradling a tiny pink bundle. She leaned forward so I could see what was in the pink blanket she was holding. It was obviously a baby but this was not right, we were expecting a boy, in a blue blanket

I would have thought. Why was she showing me this baby?

"Meet your son". I looked properly now as the words she had just said registered in my tired brain. The moment I looked at him it was as if there was nothing else in the world that mattered. I stared into his tiny crumpled face as the nurse handed him to me still in my sitting position. I held him in my arms and looked into his eyes. Even though he was just a few minutes old he was looking back at me. He knew who I was. He knew I was his father, we bonded immediately. For the first time in my life at the grand old age of 38 I was totally and utterly overwhelmed with emotion. I could not speak or look up at her as I was transfixed to this tiny helpless human being. From the very first seconds of seeing my son I knew without doubt that there could never be a love so intense. I knew from this point that my whole life had taken on new meaning. Everything that had passed before had been leading to this moment in time. All the pain Trudie and I had suffered was for this moment and did not matter anymore. I stroked his cheeks. I touched his hair, great black curls of it. I looked in wonderment at his tiny little hands that were barely big enough to grip my finger. I held him closely to me, I sniffed him. I cried.

I kissed his face and cried some more as my heart felt as though it might burst with joy and an intensity of love that up until now I had never thought possible.

The Birth (Part Two!)   165

I knew without doubt that from this point until the day I died there would be nothing I would not do to protect and care for my son.

'I'm not sure if I even want a baby', these were the words I had uttered to Trudie many years ago. If only I knew then what I would be experiencing now. Trudie had known all along that the years of striving for this moment would be so worth it and I have thanked her ever since for giving me the best thing that has ever happened in my life.

I stood up holding my son close and looking towards the theatre doors asked the nurse how Trudie was. Before she could reply the doors swung open and I got my answer. She was on a bed being wheeled out to go back onto the ward. I could see she had been heavily sedated but even through the medication she was attempting to sit up to see the precious bundle I was holding. The entourage stopped momentarily so that I could introduce mother and son. Trudie smiled weakly and slowly put out her hand to touch her baby and was trying to say something. She looked confused. She later told me that like me she saw the pink blanket the baby was wrapped in and presumed she had a girl.

Boy, girl, mongoose with yellow stripes - to either of us it did not matter one jot. We had finally reached the end of a very long and turbulent journey. A journey on which we had laughed and cried often. A journey on which we learned so much about each other, our strength's and weaknesses, hopes and aspirations. A journey on which we learned to support each other in everything we do. A journey on which we realised down the years that the best people to rely on in any given circumstance was each other and we still abide by that philosophy today.

Life is all about journeys where we experience different things. Highs and lows, happiness and sadness, challenges and achievements. We both knew that although we had come a long, long way our toughest test lay ahead of us in the years to come. Being parents is not just about giving birth then sitting back on your laurels it's about giving your child the best of yourself in every way you can. It does not matter if you are a billionaire or a pauper you owe it to your child to be the best that you can be.

Outside influences will always test your resolve to be the best parents you can be. Outside the nucleus of the family unit there are so many factors that challenge each of us on a daily basis. Living in the 21st century has its positives and negatives.

On the positive side of things medical science gave us our dream of having a child through IVF. It may have taken 12 long years but we got there eventually and we are not alone in benefiting from the wonders of science as thousands of couples each year realise their dreams of starting a family as we did. Yes there are thousands more who are unsuccessful but so were we. 144 times unsuccessful and we say to anyone who finds themselves in our situation, don't ever give up. Keep on trying and believing!

Fact is after 6 failed IVF treatments we believed we had reached the end of the road as our money ran out and we no longer qualified for treatment on the NHS.

It was Trudie's mum and step-dad, who offered to pay for the final treatment, the one that worked. Trudie refused their help in the first instance but they convinced her to accept the financial assistance they were offering. They did not want paying back, they were simply being the 'best that they could be as parents' and over the years they have been paid back tenfold. Not in cash but through the special bond that both of them now have with their grandson.

Money or lack of it played a big part in our IVF. It was not that we did not earn reasonable salaries over the years but the fact we must have spent around £35k on various treatments over time. Yes it's a hell of a lot of money but you only need to meet our son and see the happiness he spreads around him on a daily basis to know that every penny was well spent.

You could be forgiven for thinking that we were now in a position to move on financially and get our lives back on track. However the negatives of living in the 21st century were still ahead of us and any money worries we thought we had before paled into insignificance as we were to experience the effects of the global financial crash first-hand with potentially devastating effect.

Blokes

Lloyd:

I find most 'blokes' like to talk about themselves and boast about their exploits usually in a much exaggerated way following a few pints of ale. This bragging can take on many shapes and forms but generally speaking the list of topics to 'big yourself up' on is limited to two, namely 'sexual prowess' and 'earnings capability'. Of course there are many sub-headings that can sit quite comfortably under these and you could hear such as, "Yes I have a wonderful family", meaning, 'Have you seen how fit my wife is? Yep I pulled her', or "didn't I produce spectacular kids from my grade A sperm?" Or, "Oh I make big decisions for one of the top Investment Banks in the City" ... read as 'I earn shit loads of money!'

It's very blokey to draw attention to the things we feel make us look even blokier while on the other hand most guys will steer well clear of any conversation that may question in anyway their ability to produce offspring and then of course the ability to provide for them financially.

Anyone casting doubt on their blokeyness in this way is a bad person to be avoided at all cost and meaningful conversation with these people is a definite no no!

It may sound as if I'm generalising rather a lot here and it's all too easy to claim that the majority of guys are more than happy to hold the bragging rights on subjects they believe make them look good both to other blokes and the opposite sex while totally submerging anything that could be questioning their very fragile testosterone levels but I'm speaking from experience here.

Speaking from the experience of having been that loud mouthed drunk claiming to be a millionaire sex god but also the experience of being the guy who often breaks the mould as I freely and openly discuss my feelings and fears on the same topics when potentially I'm not going to look very good at all.

So what's the big deal then? What's wrong in guys doing what guys do or in this case don't do i.e. getting all 'girly' and talking about how we really feel be it good or bad? The big deal is that lack of communication can often have far more reaching consequences than we might imagine and this is where the girls get it right, far more than we do.

Women seem to have cottoned on to the idea that it's good to talk, usually to other women, (probably because blokes to talk to are in short supply). Be it a best friend, mother, sister etc. they don't do all that bottling up stuff that guys tend to think is necessary in order to preserve their masculinity. Women find someone who will listen then set about offloading. It's like therapy where a second opinion or alternative viewpoint more often than not simply confirms what they actually thought in the first place but at least they have been through a process of rationalisation that gives them the confidence to take whatever action is needed in order to resolve their problems.

Us guys need to follow suit in times of trouble because we don't cope nearly as well as we like to think we do. When was the last time you heard that a woman had slaughtered her family before killing herself and then when the evidence is unravelled it becomes clear that money worries were at the heart of the problem? I'm very well read and keep up with news and current affairs but can't recall such a scenario. On the other hand however, numerous similar incidents spring to mind where men have perpetrated such mayhem.

In the past week there has been a news story where a man has killed his wife and two beautiful daughters in their home before hanging himself! Follow up reports go on to reveal that he was up to his eyes in debt, a lot of it tragically was as a result of many years paying for IVF treatment. It also transpires that he had been in an IVA situation that clearly was not working for him.

When the initial story broke I was genuinely shocked at what I read and heard - who wouldn't be? When I read a couple of days later that a lot of the debt was run up paying for IVF treatment and the guy had been in an IVA a chill ran down my spine. It made me think that his situation seemed eerily similar to mine just a couple of years ago. I never knew him or his family but feel so sorry for them and the loved ones left behind. What state of mind must he have been in to carry out such an extreme act? In his rationale he must have arrived at the conclusion that it was best way out for all concerned!

One of my first thoughts was 'who did he speak to?' I can only presume no one because otherwise there would have been signs, someone would have seen the danger signals but apparently there were none.

Okay the vast majority of men who experience fertility and or financial problems like this don't arrive at the conclusion that such a tragic outcome is the only option open to them but there are still far too many avoidable instances of men taking their own lives, or families breaking up all for the want of sitting down with someone and opening up to them. Talking through your problems does not mean you are weak. Seeking a second opinion or asking for advice or just needing a sounding board shows you are strong. It shows you are meeting your problems head on and looking for a solution, a way forward.

As I said, women find this a lot easier to do than men and I can think of a number of instances closer to home where Trudie and I have had to watch, helpless, while friends of ours have split up from seemingly great relationships and every time it's because the guy in these relationships has refused to talk about their problems.

They say that if you are an alcoholic you can't start to heal yourself until you outwardly acknowledge you have a problem and I believe that's the same with lots of issues we face in life. No, I'm not saying you have to attend meetings with other people in a similar situation then stand up and proclaim "I'm Lloyd and I'm a Bankrupt" or, "I'm Lloyd and I cant have children", but we do need to go through some sort of process of speaking to someone who is not immediately affected by the situation. Where we accept the position we are in and show that we will not be influenced or intimidated by what other people may think to the negative. After all, the people that really matter to you will surely help and support you far more than you maybe realise and these are the people you need to speak to.

Of course there will always be those who take some sort of sick satisfaction from your plight but what are they to you anyway? Does it really matter what they think? Do you really care? Care about what your loved ones think of you because they will always see the good in you as a person and will want to help.

I'm not meaning to have a downer on guys here because I think the reluctance to speak out and share a problem is inbuilt, it's in our makeup but we do need to go against our natural instincts of quietly getting on with it sometimes. I don't exaggerate when I say Trudie and I have seen many relationships end in separation when there were other potential outcomes if only the guy in the relationship had been prepared to say his piece be it good or bad.

It's not a time for men to be the 'strong, silent type', trust me guys, you need to talk about your fears and anxieties in order to relieve some of the pressure you are under. I can't help thinking that if all these men are out there not talking to each other, then the chances of them speaking to the women in their lives are probably remote too?

There is always the exception to every rule and just to prove the point I can tell you about another guy I know who through IVF had twin boys. He and his wife were in treatment a couple of years after we had Jayjay. This guy is typical of the loud, over confident boaster following a couple of pints I referred to earlier. I used to work with him and he began to tentatively ask me the odd question here and there as to how we eventually conceived Jayjay? I would always just answer his questions without seeking more information because I thought if he wanted to talk then that was up to him. It soon became apparent that his questions were far more than just idle interest and in fact he and his wife were having fertility treatment.

I was talking one night to Trudie about it and she thought his questions were maybe an invite for me to respond to him in more depth, maybe he just didn't know how to broach the subject properly. I thought she's probably right, maybe he does want to really pick my brains but is afraid to ask. Next time he raises the subject I'll help him out.

What a mistake that was! It wasn't long after when we were in the pub one Friday after work and again following a couple of drinks he was asking me about Trudie and Jayjay and how long it had taken us to conceive him through fertility treatment? I responded by asking him outright if he and his wife were on IVF? The answer I got knocked me right back, "Are we fuck on IVF. Who told you that pile of shit?" I wasn't offended or embarrassed by this but I was certainly embarrassed for him. I knew they were on IVF. He knows I knew they were on IVF, yet his manly insecurities would not allow him to admit it regardless of how stupid he was looking.

Since then I still see him and his kids around as they live locally but conversation is very brief particularly if there are other people around. It's as if he fears me coming up to him and saying something like, "Hi how are you and your wonderful IVF children?" Yes, even after all these years he won't admit that they needed a little help from medical science in order to realise their dreams of having a family. It's as if he's ashamed in some way and I wonder if he's told the kids the wonderful and special circumstances in which they came in to this world or will they, like him, grow up believing that 'silence is golden'?

We have told our son all about the IVF years, the highs and the lows, the patience, anguish and dedication it took to get him and he tells us how special it makes him feel knowing how much we wanted him. Best of all is how he communicates his feelings to us, his grandparents, his friends and teachers; in fact anyone he believes has an alternative viewpoint to the one he holds. He's not necessarily looking for answers all the time because he is a very confident young guy capable of making his own decisions but he's already cottoned onto the idea that talking and communicating can help us all through all manner of difficult situations that may arise in our lives.

Better

Homes

Trudie:

"Mrs Trudie Thompson?" came the voice on the other end of the line,

"Yes?" I tentatively confirmed.

"Hi my names Joy, I am the producer on 'Better Homes' the TV programme……"

I didn't hear anything further, my mind was a blank, someone was playing a wicked joke.

"Mrs Thompson, are you there?" enquired the voice.

"Yes!" I stammered, "And yes I know of the programme" I quickly added as I didn't want her to think me rude. I'd wanted to be on Better Homes since the show began, but I was still wondering if someone was having a laugh at my expense but also not wanting to alienate Joy if she really was who she said she was so I carried on, "It's one of my favourite shows, I've watched every series a hundred times". Everyone knew 'Better Homes'. Excitement surged through my bones and I was visibly shaking, 'oh my God'. I could hardly breathe.

"Were you aware that your husband had written to us?"

I was well aware Lloyd had written to them though I'd never actually seen the letter. He had started on his quest to repay me for my perseverance when Jayjay was first born. I cast my mind back and distinctly remembered a day when passing the lounge to take some washing upstairs, I overheard a conversation that made me want to burst with love.

Lloyd was busy feeding our wonderful new son who was only a few weeks old. He'd thrown him over his shoulder in order to burp him as this was the most comfortable way for Lloyd due to him only having the use of one arm. I remember that he was stood gazing out of the front room window whilst gently patting Jayjay's tiny back. He was swaying too and fro and lovingly explaining that Jayjay was probably the luckiest baby alive as he had the best mummy in the world, the type of mummy that Carlsberg would produce if they could.

"Your mummy spent her life believing in her dream and against all the odds she just kept on keeping on and kept on believing. Mummy is very inspirational, one day I shall find a way to repay her for bringing you to us. She is so clever, she knew how much I would love and adore you, even when I was totally discouraged and disheartened and didn't know whether I wanted to be someone's dad, how smart is that? Your good old mum just kept on believing. She kept telling me to trust her and that I would not only make the best dad but I would marvel in and enjoy every ounce of it. Oh how right she was. She's the best Jay and we're the lucky ones." I stopped on the stairs and listened. Lloyd unaware of my presence just carried on singing my praises and saying all the things that every mother deserves to hear and not just because she covered 12 years on infertility but just because us mum's deserve to hear it.

By this time happy tears were cascading down my cheeks onto the washing I had cradled in my arms.

How lucky was I, this was most definitely a moment I'd cherish for as long as I lived.

So, yes I was well aware that my lovely husband had written to Better Homes as he was frantically trying to find a way to thank me. He'd told me that he'd written to them but that all seemed so long ago now.

I could hear Joy's breath and was unsure how long I'd drifted; I came back to earth and managed a measly, "Yes".

"Excellent, that makes my job so much easier, and I'm pleased to inform you that you are down to the final 25".

25 what? I thought, and as if reading my mind Joy carried on… "We have chosen 25 out of the 25,000 applications". Wow I had no idea so many people wrote in. Joy was still speaking, "Please don't get your hopes too high because we visit each couple, carry out an interview on camera then we decide which houses/people to choose for this series".

It became apparent that they only required 8 homes, so making it to 25 probably wasn't that big a deal. Still it was nice to speak to someone famous.

It was arranged that the crew would visit the following Monday and our instructions were to act as normally as possible!

I could not wait to tell Lloyd.

He was completely gob smacked and he brought me the letter he'd written on the 9th June 2001 which read…

"Dear Carol

Having watched your programme for the past few years, I decided to put pen to paper and beg your expertise.

I met Trudie, my lovely wife some 17 years ago and we have been happily married for the last 15 years. 3 years ago we bought the house of our dreams, a Victorian semi-detached with all the trimmings, huge hallway, tall ceilings etc. even a 100-year-old chandelier. It was just perfect; it needed plenty of work but nonetheless perfect – just see the enclosed Estate Agents details, it just knocked our socks off!

Anyway, we spent many years on fertility treatment (12 to be precise) and we didn't hold out much hope of ever becoming parents but we plodded on, as you do, then we found our dream home. At first we ummed and arghed about whether to buy it (because of the cost of renovation) but in the end we just threw ourselves into it in a very haphazard way, probably hoping it would comfort our sorrows.

To cut a very long story short, our very last IVF treatment worked and we now have the most wonderful little boy, Jayjay (an African name meaning 'most precious gift from God') – how lucky are we? House of our dreams and now a child! We had so many plans when we first saw the house and moved in, but unfortunately all we have managed to accomplish to date, now that we have Jayjay, is utter confusion and we desperately need your help.

Trudie has just registered as a child minder (having been a legal secretary all her life), and we would dearly love to have the attic converted into some sort of play area to try and preserve the rest of the house. Also we are in dire need of a new bathroom; the one we have is literally falling off the walls. But really we would dearly love your comments and input, we have so many ideas but they've all become somewhat jumbled – a bit like this letter.

Anyway rather than chunner on relentlessly it would be an absolute dream come true if you could come and take a look and consider us as this would be the ideal way to say a huge THANK YOU to Trudie for persevering all those years and making me a Dad.

Well I've done all I can do, but I am a true believer in the saying "if you don't raise your hand you can't be counted" – so here I am raising my hand and I thank you in great anticipation of being counted.

Yours extremely hopefully etc. etc. etc."

Wow, I was blown away, it was no wonder Better Homes were considering us, I was married to a genius, I threw my arms around him and I knew at that very moment that we would be one of the 8 that Joy had spoken about.

The days passed and Monday galloped towards us. What would we wear? What should we say? How nervous were we? It was all well and good Joy saying 'just be natural' how on earth do you do that knowing that if you're chosen Carol Vorderman would come to your home! Surreal!

'Come on NATURAL/NORMAL don't fail us now'.

"They're here", called Lloyd from the front room. Jayjay hadn't a clue what was going on, all he knew was we had visitors and boy did Jayjay love having visitors, the more the merrier. He'd always been very sociable and he ran to the door where his daddy was meeting and greeting folk. One more check in the mirror, lippy OK, and deep breath and away we go. "And this is my lovely wife Trudie", gestured Lloyd as a bevy of beauties graced the hallway.

Joy quickly put us at our ease and we went into the living room. We chatted about the years on IVF and how we'd met each other. Jayjay was an angel often stealing the show with his cheeky repartee and everyone fell in love with him as everyone always did. The time passed quickly and it wasn't as nerve racking as you'd imagine. As they departed Joy said we would be contacted in the near future once they had made their decisions. So now it was just a waiting game. We were used to that, we'd spent our lives waiting, waiting for doctors appointments, waiting for results, waiting just waiting, so this we knew we could do.

We didn't need to wait too long. The following week I was at play group with Jay when my mobile phone rang. It was Joy. It was very loud in the play area so my friend watched Jay whilst I nipped to the Ladies to take the call in peace.

"Hi Trudie its Joy",

"Hiya",

"I won't beat about the bush, YOU'RE IN".

You could have knocked me down with a feather. I was going on Better Homes. More to the point, Carol Vorderman was coming to my house. Joy carried on.

"You've got George Bond as your designer".

I was struggling to take it all in. George Bond, the GEORGE BOND, was going to design my 3-bed semi in Leyland. Fantastic! Wonderful! I needed to get off the phone because I needed to ring Lloyd. I needed to get back to the play group and bellow so all the world would know.

We discussed the process from that stage. Not that I could concentrate but I got the gist. All I could imagine was Carol Vorderman and George Bond, I could not believe my luck. I have always said that I truly am the luckiest person alive and this just confirmed my belief, anything I wanted I got. First there was the lovely Lloyd, then there was our precious baby and now the house of our dreams was to be renovated by the magnificent George Bond. I was all a quiver; I had huge butterflies in my stomach. My heart raced at twice its normal speed and I felt as though I was permanently walking on air.

The weeks went by and all manner of people visited, they would measure this and that and they would enquire as to our likes and dislikes. We were given two boards, one was called a 'love board' where we were to put pictures of all the things we loved, colours, fabrics, pictures of kitchens, lounges, bedrooms, light fittings etc. etc. etc. and the other board was to be a 'hate board', where we were to paste pictures of all the things we didn't want in our home.

We loved this part and we had no idea what they were going to do. The wonderful George asked what we would do if money were no object, so obviously we took down walls, made rooms larger we would swan around our home in some kind of fantasy world and George would always indulge us, he would encourage us to dream bigger and grander. Our 'love' and 'hate' boards were full of pictures by now. We bought every home magazine that had ever been produced and we'd spent hours cutting and sticking pictures. It was fabulous.

Eventually Monday morning the 11th March 2002 arrived. This was the chosen day. This was the day that Better Homes were to move in and we were to move out. Ding dong, the front door bell rang and we all ran to answer it to find Ms Vorderman gracing our step. Why oh why were we all so surprised? She was wonderful, she obviously sensed how nervous we were as we stood there jostling for her attention and lets face it she'd been filming Better Homes for a number of years therefore she had met many people who would have felt the way we did at this moment. We quickly invited her in and I remember making tea and chatting as though we'd known her forever. Carol Vorderman in my house at 8am on a Monday morning who'd have thought it?

I also remember thinking how glamorous, elegant and beautiful she was. Again I was amazed at why this should surprise me. She was so funny and so kind. I couldn't get over how tall and slim she was, the television does not do this lady justice at all.

The film crew and our production manager, Lorraine, had set up all the equipment in order to film us in our house before the makeover. They were brilliant and we felt as though we'd been TV stars all our lives. This was surely our destiny!

After filming came the part where we were to leave which felt more than a tad weird. We could only return home on the Friday for the Big Reveal. That was one heck of a long drawn out week I can tell you. It was hard to sleep. It was hard to eat. In fact it was hard to concentrate on anything at all. Though as a couple we were used to waiting this was seriously testing. What were they doing to our home and how were our neighbours dealing with the all the disruption? I knew that our neighbours would be patient as we knew them all very well. It's a lovely welcoming neighbourhood full of kind souls; we live in a community that always pulls together no matter what. Our community is the type that people write about usually in the past tense! These people want to know how you are doing, these are the people that lift your spirits and would save your soul should your soul ever need saving. I love our neighbourhood so I was truly hoping that the strangers that were very kindly re-building our home wouldn't ride rough shot over their feelings.

It was FRIDAY. We waited for that phone call, the one that would summon us home. It came. We set off immediately. As we rounded the corner we could not believe our eyes, the whole of Leyland, well the whole world in fact, had turned out to welcome us, they were waving, clapping and cheering. Jayjay wasn't sure about his new found celebrity status and quickly buried his head in my neck. Carol and Lorraine met us at the corner shop and through all the din and mayhem; they began to talk us through the next stage. We approached the house with the whole world watching. Carol guided us as we had to keep our eyes shut. This was it. The cameras were already rolling as they need to catch our initial reaction. This was a one time moment. There could be no retakes and there was no going back.

I heard Carol start her 'piece to camera'. My heart was thumping and as usual I was hanging onto Lloyd's hand. I could feel my chin quiver and tears were already escaping my closed eyelids and dripping off my cheeks. Carol was reading our story, our whole story. The story of how we'd arrived at this moment in our lives and I stood there listening intently to the familiar events and awaiting the queue to open our eyes and take in our new surroundings. My chin quivered on and my eyes wouldn't dry up and embarrassment of all embarrassments my nose was now running. What a lovely way to greet the nation, mascara all over and snot hanging off my nose, classy bird or what?

It was then I heard Carol's warm voice utter, "Open your eyes", I could not have dreamt in my wildest dreams what met my vision. All I remember of that blurry moment in time was turning to Carol and mouthing the words, "Do we get to keep it?" And after that I was lost for words! I believe Carol cried too.

Our home was beautiful, as you'd imagine, George had truly excelled in his brilliance as one of the nations top designers he most definitely, without a shadow of a doubt, is the best of the best and we are eternally grateful to everyone who had a hand in fulfilling yet another dream.

I sometimes look around my life and I am always amazed at the miracles that occur on a daily basis.

From Retail to Finance

Lloyd:

I'm not quite sure when the need to earn as much money as I possibly could took over from my, until then, belief that I should work to live not live to work. Maybe it was the fact that IVF was proving to be a very costly process over the years that made me move away from an industry that I loved into one that was relatively rather dull but gave me the opportunity to earn a lot more cash.

Working in 'fashion retail' was the perfect job for me. Great clothes and music playing all day while meeting new people. I didn't consider my job as work; it was more like a night out without the drinking and dancing. I tell a lie there, as many a time I would have a little bit of a groove on the shop floor if a tune grabbed me.

I started in retail at the age of 18 and had a successful career working for various national companies. I was good at what I did purely because it all came naturally to me and I was doing what I wanted to do. I was not a slave to my job or any organisation that I worked for.

I also ran my own business in the early 90s when I realised a long standing ambition and opened an 'up market' menswear boutique of my own. I'll spare you the detail but suffice to say we got our first taste of how things can go horrendously wrong when the financial side of things goes belly up. We closed the shop and lost £22k of our own money that had been invested in the project. It was a hell of a lot of money then and really tested our ability to bounce back both financially and as a couple.

We were in the relatively early years of our IVF treatments and having our own business was supposed to be a means to earning the sort of money we wanted to fund our IVF while enjoying the lifestyle we were accustomed to. We got first hand experience of how the big banks in this country work when they believe they are at risk of losing money. We saw how relentless they can be when pursuing individuals for money they are owed. Any avenue will be considered by the Banks if it means recovering the debt. In our case it was the crazy offer of even more money to 'bolster the business'.

"Your shop is a sound business Mr and Mrs Thompson, you are simply in need of a boost to your cash flow and the bank is prepared to lend you up to £20k".

The offer was tempting but together we were strong and rational and decided it was best to cut our losses and clear the debts we already had with the bank. It did however open our eyes to the irresponsible way that banks were prepared to throw money around to people who would not be able to pay it back.

Once we refused the offer of further funding we saw a different side to the 'friendly face of banking' as our bank manager did a 'Jekyll & Hyde' and started making ludicrous demands for repayment of monies owed and threatening us with this penalty and that charge, as if he were attacking us with his financial machete.

However, we stayed strong - as we always do - and managed to clear the debt inside 12 months, our lifestyle taking a temporary setback as we lived on beans and toast and Trudie took on an extra job to bring in more money. Suffice to say fertility treatment had to sit on the back-burner while we sorted ourselves out.

The fact we were able to clear our debts without incurring any defaults or CCJ's was to prove incredibly and ironically significant just a couple of years later when I joined the world of Financial Services.

You may be wondering how someone who has sold clothing all their working years suddenly ends up as a 'financial adviser' then ultimately a manager of a lending bank? Well, it gives you a bit of an insight into what our banks really do. I was approached by a recruitment consultant who was working for one of the 'Big Five' as they were known at that time. It mattered not one jot if you had no experience of financial services. What they were looking for were 'sales people', and I had been a salesman all my life. The bank was finding it easier to recruit sales people and teach them the financial side of the job than to teach bankers how to sell.

It's rather scary to think that the big national banks were prepared to recruit on such criteria. It was almost as if having the financial experience hardly mattered as long as you had the 'gift of the gab', the ability to persuade people to borrow money or take out insurance policies they hardly needed. Yes, I took and passed all the necessary exams to allow me to do my job but I will say now - hand on heart - I never really knew 100% what I was doing and know people still working in the industry today who are by no means experts in their role.

The banks are more interested in sitting their customers in front of someone who can persuade them to take out a loan and all the add-on income generators such as 'payment protection' as opposed to giving their customers sound financial advice. They take advantage of people who are in desperate financial straits who can be easily manipulated by the situation they find themselves in. I look back now and realise that I joined 'the enemy'. Less than two years after our own disputes with the bank here I was earning a living throwing money at people who should not have been borrowing as they were always likely to struggle to pay it back. Yes, they met all the bank's criteria and ticked all the right boxes but many a time I knew as I sat face to face with these individuals that I was signing them up for a bag-load of trouble.

I am ashamed of the job I used to do and the only thing I would say in my defence is that I was always working within the lending criteria of the bank. If the computer said yes, I was duty bound to lend the money. The lending targets of the bank were very demanding and only outweighed by the demands to collect the bad debts that were subsequently incurred as the customers got themselves into the vicious circle of borrowing and debt.

The whole process of 'collecting' arrears and bad debt is like a military operation in itself. If the lenders put as much effort into finding out the real circumstances of their clients before dishing out the dosh, as they do in attempting to recoup their losses, it would save everyone a lot of trouble and aggravation. Trust me when I say they will leave no stone unturned as they delve into every little aspect of your life to discover what you earn, where you earn it, who you are paying out to, who else you are in arrears with and so on. They want to know all this stuff because anyone else that you owe money to suddenly becomes 'a competitor'. They want your cash. They don't want the other bank down the road getting his pound of flesh before they get theirs.

The 'collection centres' working for the banking organisations are absolutely ruthless in their pursuit of your last penny. You stop being a customer and in their eyes turn into 'the scum of the earth' who have dared to miss an instalment or two on loan repayments.

Whole armies of people are employed to sit in call centres ringing 'bad debtors', chasing you for money that you don't have. Believe it or not the rule of not ringing you at work goes completely out of the window when you are in a debt situation, and it's completely legal for the creditors to try and track you down via work as long as they do not break the data protection laws and many a thin ice is skated on there.

I know all this because I have worked in that environment. I can honestly say I always treated people with the dignity that any human being deserves, but both Trudie and I have been on the receiving end of some of the most unscrupulous and callous individuals you could come across, attempting to bully you into submission by threatening all manner of consequences for not paying up. It does not stop with phone calls and threatening letters either. When they decide to turn up the heat under you, debt collectors can come knocking at your door.

One pathetic individual actually saw fit to hand a 'letter of demand' to my then nine-year-old son to 'pass onto his Daddy'. Luckily for this character Trudie was in while I was at work so all he got was a flea in his ear, as opposed to having his lights punched out for doing that to my little boy. And I am by no means a violent man.

For years I earned a handsome living getting people into debt, as the banks pay great commissions and bonuses on the back of the billions of pounds they make from lending. However, in years to come I would see the whole scenario from the other side of the fence as a bankrupt myself.

My experience of working for 'the enemy' was to prove invaluable in those later years as I fought for my financial life. Knowing how the banks work and being a former insider was the ace up my sleeve as my creditors tried to turn me into just another statistic on the financial junk heap.

Bodyform
For You!

Lloyd:

At face value the financial and legal systems of this country appear to be well regulated by bodies such as the Financial Services Authority, various Ombudsmen and of course the Government themselves. There are supposed to be rules, regulations and systems in place to ensure that the flow of money and finances in our banking network is fair and regulated and ensure that individuals are not put at risk of accruing bad debt and or losing their home and possessions.

In other words banks, credit card companies and finance houses have a duty to carry out what's known as 'responsible lending', meaning they should always have the customers' 'best interest' at the forefront of their actions, even if that means not lending money is the best thing for the customer on the basis that they will struggle to pay it back.

The regulatory bodies also have the same obligations in their approach to recovering bad debts. Yes, monies lent that are in arrears need to be collected but as ever the customer should be treated the right way, particularly as in so many cases these days the lender has been culpable in aiding and abetting the debt situation.

At face value everything is legally in place to ensure that we have a fair and just financial system where everyone is doing the right thing and applying the letter of the law in every case. And if you do happen to get into debt then surely it must be your fault entirely. At least that's what the money people would have us believe anyway.

Having worked in numerous financial institutions down the years and then had the misfortune to end up in a cul-de-sac myself I have taken a step back in order to analyse what really goes on in the world of finance and what I find is really scary. It's almost as if all the companies who lend money, collect bad debts or run bad debt programmes have formed a cartel whereby once you are unfortunate enough to fall off the slippery slope and end up in debt then they have you trapped in the system forever. Unless you have your wits about you.

Let me explain by taking the example of some of the big finance companies out there. I don't have to name names because you know the sort of organisations I mean. They advertise daily via our TV screens, although I still fail to understand why they believe their target audience is sat at home glued to the box in the middle of the day. Surely we're all out at work, or maybe you don't need to hold down a job these days to obtain finance. One of the bigger companies even has its own TV channel, for crying out loud! I know that TV advertising is not cheap and it shows the lengths the finance companies will go in order to seduce us into applying to them for money or debt management. Their polished glitzy ads show us how we could be enjoying blue skies and sandy beaches in faraway countries, pretty much along the lines of an advert a few years ago for female sanitary products showing a girl being pulled along a golden sea front on roller skates by her dog. She looked to be having such a wonderful time that I wanted to have periods and use their product if it meant life would be so good. Well that's the same principle on which the money lenders are working. They know that the people likely to take notice of their ads are more often than not in dire straits, and therefore easily seduced by the images and promises they broadcast. In the first instance they are offering to put a protective arm around you and lend you that money or erase your debt in order to sort out your miserable life forever. They will convince you that you are more than capable of making your repayments. And that's easy for them to do because when you are backed into a corner you are easy prey and will believe anything they tell you, because you want to.

But hang on a minute, why would any right-minded business person lend money to anyone who may not be able to pay it back? That would be stupid and a fast track way to business ruination, wouldn't it? Yet this is where the plot thickens.

Lending you that money is a risk but it's a risk they are prepared to take because best case scenario is that you do pay it back in full and on time and the lender makes a handsome profit courtesy of the extortionate interest rate you signed up for when you were blinded by the sunlight from the glowing sea front in the advert.

However, if you can't pay back the money they still have no reason to worry. Why? Because they now have you on the first rung of the ladder. You are well and truly on-board the financial merry-go-round whereby they can make money out of your situation regardless of which way you turn from this point on.

Do you know that it's common practice for one and the same company to be lending, collecting, doing debt management and practising in IVA's? Sometimes, all from the same premises. What's wrong with that? What's wrong is that in every process listed above there is commission to be made, money to be earned from you. The lender makes big bucks via your interest repayments and any late fees you may accrue, collection companies earn commission according to how much they collect, debt management generates commission and the IVA practitioners charge for their services. No matter how it may be dressed up - be it fees, commission, interest or whatever - it comes out of your pocket. There are no free lunches in finance.

I'm not making this up either. I have worked for numerous companies where the full spectrum of financial services are available to you. With that in mind surely the whole ethos of 'responsible lending' can be brought into question. After all, if I'm lending you money that ultimately it transpires you can't afford to pay back in full, I'm not going to worry too much. I will have made some profit up to the point you go into default. Then when I pass you on to my debt management department I'll make more from you there. Once you realise that under debt management you are still getting hassle from other creditors I'll move you onto an IVA, where I will continue to make money off the back of your financial plight. Surely not, I hear you saying. But it's true, it's what goes on. These companies even make money by selling your name to other companies to offer services to. I have witnessed people buying and selling lists of names (leads) of people in debt for thousands of pounds for the potential rewards that can be gained once they manage to get their claws into you.

At one place I used to work in Manchester it was common practice for the guys selling loans to pass customers straight through to the debt management department in the rare instances they could not lend. And they received commission for each one they passed across because they were keeping the customer on the merry-go-round! The guys tasked with collecting arrears would do the same.

The sad thing is that these companies continue to get away with it because they can blind us with science and complicated jargon, knowing we are desperate to find a solution to our problems. We get blinded to the fact that we are being passed around and squeezed for more and more money that we just don't have.

In my own situation, having lost my business and realising practically overnight that drastic measures were needed to fix my finances I thought an IVA would be the solution. I owed £100k to banks, credit cards and car finance. I took the responsible step of notifying all my creditors immediately, working on the premise that they would understand and look favourably on the fact that I was being up front about my circumstances and not hiding from anyone. The IVA company I opted to go with were making all the right noises. "Oh, we'll take care of everything, we'll keep your creditors off your back, just refer anyone chasing you for money straight through to us". An ideal solution under the circumstances you would think, but it turned out to be nothing of the sort because everyone in the system is after just one thing - your money. Even when they realise you are on the bones of your backside they want to get as big a share as they can before the next guy gets his.

The people you owe money to don't ease up on you as they continue to chase and harass you day and night. The IVA company I had used which was one of the biggest and most 'reputable' in the country, appeared incapable of managing the situation. And it was after 5 months, during which time I had paid them nearly four grand, it transpired that not one penny had been paid to any of my creditors. They gave excuses about not having all the settlement figures they needed in order to start apportioning payments, and the first three monthly payments by me were allocated to their fees. No wonder I was still getting hassle from my creditors. The IVA company that were purporting to be my financial salvation had actually got me into more debt and arrears than I had before I ever spoke to them.

I then considered getting a solicitor involved, but dismissed the idea on the grounds that I would simply be bringing another party to the merry-go-round to take more money off me.

I realised that if I was to get out of the mess I was in, then I would have to apply the old adage of 'if you want something doing properly, then do it yourself'. So that's what I did.

When you start to look for it there is so much help and advice available for people who are in a mess with their money. There is the Citizens Advice Bureau where you can talk to someone 'for free'. There is the 'Consumer Credit Counselling Service' that can help you, again for free. There are all sorts of booklets and pamphlets explaining different options such as IVA's, debt management and bankruptcy, and in this age of the internet you can find enough online to keep you busy for months.

I know I had an advantage with my financial background and it gave me the confidence to go it alone. But all the information available is purposely made easy to understand. Anyone of reasonable intelligence should be able to work out what's best for their situation without having to spend more money they don't have paying someone to do a job they can do themselves.

Entering into an IVA and paying nearly £4,000 into a scheme that ultimately did not work for me was a costly exercise, and I'm sure it's a scenario that's played out on numerous other occasions with other vulnerable people across the land everyday. My advice is to explore every avenue open to you before you start paying out to solicitors or IVA companies. Read every leaflet and pamphlet and speak to every person you can who is offering free advice before deciding on your next course of action.

While you are finding your way forward you need to be strong and stick up for yourself when your creditors are threatening you with all manner of dire consequences, because most of the time they are just threats designed to make you find the money to pay them from somewhere.

Above all, never pay out to credit card companies or to loans at the expense of not paying your mortgage! No court in the land would support anyone trying to get money out of you to address unsecured debts if it meant you were putting at risk the roof over your family's heads. In 30 years of being a house owner I have never missed a single mortgage payment and consequently my mortgage company treats me very well in spite of my current financial status.

Think about it. If you are on-side with your mortgage company and know your home is safe, what can these other creditors really threaten you with? If you take time out to do an honest, detailed income expenditure and offer a fair and reasonable amount towards your debts, what can they do to you? Come round and knee-cap you? Abduct your kids? No they will use scary words like 'default' and 'CCJ' in the hope that you will offer them more than you can afford. Remember be strong and stick up for yourself, because there are bigger and scarier words out there, and even then it's never as bad as you think. I know because it was the route I eventually decided to take for myself.

Bankruptcy

Lloyd:

When I had been told that I had to 'go to Court', I never for one moment thought it would be a real court. I thought I would be in an office-type scenario speaking to some guy in a suit discussing my finances, something similar to the hundreds of 'business meetings' I had been in over the years, a situation I would be familiar and comfortable with. How wrong could I have been? Yep. It was a real court I was attending and I was sitting in a real court waiting room, waiting to be called in to face a real judge!

The guy with the bad body odour on my right had sat down far too close for comfort, while the dishevelled individual immediately on my left could have been sat 10 yards away and his pungent beer breath would still have been making my eyes water! OK, you're thinking, a bloke's allowed to have a drink. But this was 10.30 in the morning!

The court appearances were obviously running late so I took time out to scan the room and observe the different characters around me. There must have been 30 or so people in there and the majority of them made me think that the judges would be spending the whole day thumping down their gavels and proclaiming most of them 'guilty'. I don't usually jump to conclusions and 'judge' books by their cover, but you didn't need to be a genius to see the room was filled in the main with 'low-life ne'er-do-wells'

There were however a few lost souls who looked completely out of place in this room. They did not have tattoos all over the place, or if they did they were spelt correctly. They were not arguing or pacing up and down staring people out or having loud aggressive calls on mobiles. They were not covered in cuts or bruises and sporting black eyes. I have never seen such a collection of black eyes in one place. I felt like I was attending a meeting of the Preston underworld and I, like the handful of others I had picked out, was totally out of place here.

I watched as various solicitors and barristers came and went and people came in and out of the small meeting rooms that led off from the main waiting area that I was in. I started to play a game in my head, 'match the alleged crook to the alleged crime'. I then started to wonder if any of the few individuals who looked out of place were guilty of the same crime as me... the crime of bankruptcy.

Yes I know it's not a criminal offence to go bust, so why did I have to be sharing this room with the cast of 'Fraggle Rock'? Why was I having to play the part of an extra in an episode of 'The Bill'? I don't scare easily but today I was scared. Trudie had desperately wanted to come with me as support, but right now I was so glad that I had managed to convince her that it was best if I came alone. I did not want to think of her in this environment.

What is it with the British legal system where money crime is concerned anyway? Often you hear of cases where someone has fiddled the tax man or embezzled funds from some large corporation and the perpetrator, once tried and convicted, ends up doing double the time of some creep that's been found guilty of abusing kids.

I'm not saying there were paedophiles in that room, but I still objected to being thrown in with the type of people that were there. How difficult could it be to separate a small group of people who through no fault of their own were experiencing financial difficulty, from a large group of people who in the main appeared to have opted for a life on the wrong side of the law?

As grave as the situation was, something popped into my head that made me smile. I thought of a scene from one of our favourite movies, 'Trading Places' starring Dan Aykroyd and Eddie Murphy where Aykroyd's character 'Louis Winthorpe III' finds himself in a police station having been robbed of all his wealth by unscrupulous business associates. He was a well-to-do, successful business man who'd had the dirty done on him and suddenly found himself in a seedy world that was totally alien to him. I got my mobile out and sent Trudie a text that read "I'm like Louis Winthorpe". She knew exactly what I meant, so there we were at the lowest low point in our long and eventful lives sharing joke texts about the situation we found ourselves in. Once again we were supporting each other through the hard times.

So how had it come to this? Yes I was replaying Louis Winthorpe's waiting room scene, but the similarities of my own real life journey to that courtroom were eerily and remarkably similar to his.

I suppose it had all started some 19 or so years earlier at the time I moved out of the retail fashion industry that I loved, into the world of financial services.

The time when I started to move away from my own philosophy of 'work to live' and my job started to be the overriding factor when big decisions needed to be taken. It was a necessary change in tact because I had realised I could earn a lot more managing a bank than I could managing a clothes store. It was a change I wanted to make as we were desperate to keep funding our fertility treatments, as we were now three or four years down that route and as desperate as ever to have a child. Funds were needed as we no longer qualified for free IVF treatment on the NHS. We had to find our own cash.

I'm not sure at what point I officially started to 'live to work' but it happened somewhere along the way, and I know it's certainly not something unique to me. Life has a way of demanding hard work from all of us who seek to be successful for whatever reason. Nothing is going to be handed to you on a plate, unless you are lucky enough to win the lottery. But you can't really write into your life business plan, 'Lottery win in five years' if only we could, but it ain't that easy.

I had noticed very early on in my finance career that I was working with a totally different sort of animal to my previous life. People were more driven, more money-orientated. These people were not secretive about how much they earned, in fact they wanted everyone to know how successful they were. Managers would motivate their sales people by dangling monetary carrots, by telling how much the top people were earning, "This could be you raking in £100k a year if you show the same dedication as John or Jane".

I never needed a John or a Jane to be my role model. I have my own drive and self-belief and considering I was now in a completely new environment I took to my new working life very easily. I was successful from the start and made good headway in the world of finance. So much so that I was often 'head hunted' as my reputation grew and directors of numerous organisations approached me from time to time to revamp their businesses.

Over the years it dawned on me that even though I was capable of earning good money for me and my family I was also making other individuals very rich. The directors and owners who employed me to run their companies were the ones that really benefited from my ability to 'make a business work'. Yes, I was earning big money and driving flashy company cars, but the guys at the top were making the serious dough on the back of my efforts.

Our monetary priorities had changed over the years in that we were no longer funding IVF, but we were still playing catch-up from all the years of compromising ourselves financially. Yes, we had a beautiful home but with a mortgage to match it. Down the years Trudie had been offered many jobs where she could earn much more than she did but had always refused to commit to anything which meant she could not fully concentrate on her fertility treatment.

Trudie was a legal secretary and very good at what she did, and was often tempted with jobs that could double or triple her income. But jobs like that don't come without a price. They require you to work long hours, take on stress or work away. In short, work comes before everything, and while we could certainly have done with the extra cash to fund our IVF, this was a price Trudie was not prepared to pay. It was very much a catch-22 situation because we needed the IVF to work in order to realise our dream of having a child. But if Trudie had to take some high-powered job in order to realise the dream, how would she fit it around the many appointments she needed to keep whilst on a treatment. And what would she do once the baby came along?

I often questioned Trudie's logic on this, pointing out that once we were parents she could give up working or find a low-key job, but she is a very honourable person and would never take on something that she could not see through to the end.

This is when we would come to loggerheads, and I would question whether or not our quest for parenthood would ever be fruitful or indeed roll out the old chestnut of 'I'm not sure I even want to be a dad'.

Luckily Trudie stuck to her guns in the face of my questioning and doubt. She says she always knew with undying belief that one day she would give birth to our child. And you know, I think she really did.

Down the years we had survived financially and provided the best that we could for our son, but like the majority of people surviving is just what we were doing. Not living a rip-roaring, money's-no-object kind of lifestyle. We were surviving. Yes, we managed to grab the odd holiday here and there and put decent food on the table as opposed to the beans-on-toast IVF days, but there comes a time in all our lives where we have to start thinking of securing a sound financial future for ourselves and our offspring.

We had some catching up to do as 'old' parents. We had small pensions but nowhere near enough to even provide us with the basic lifestyle in our later years, and certainly not enough to support our son in his early adult life if he was to go on to university.

He certainly was not going to inherit a mortgage-free property in the shape of the family home. The numerous remortgages we had needed down the years had seen to that. So while the now was OK and as a family we were surviving, the future looked pretty bleak. The temptation can sometimes be to bury your head in the hope that something will come along. Why worry about the future when you may never even get there? Actually that's more my philosophy than Trudie's. She does tend to worry a lot more than I do but then something did come along or certainly it seemed that way at the time.

It was three years ago when I was approached by a former employer whose business I had previously turned around. He had employed me as his 'sales director' and I had grown his company to the point where he was able to sell it, earning himself a tidy sum along the way.

This time however he was talking about us working together as partners on a business project he had based on the particular way I had organised his company for him some years earlier. There was a niche in the market that was screaming out for my original system.

He was right. There was a massive opportunity to set up a company that could capitalise on the booming financial services industry. An idea that I had developed many years ago could earn both of us a lot of money now.

Was this the break we had been hoping for? Yes as far as I was concerned, straight in there focusing on all the positives. We need to be careful, warned Trudie the ever-sensible one. Of course it looked like a fantastic proposition but we were going to have to find money to invest, very much a case of taking one step back in order to move forwards. And like I said our Mortgage was practically up to the hilt.

We discussed long into many a night all the pro's and cons.

We had been here before many years earlier of course, when we opened our boutique. And that had all ended so badly. We could have bottled it and taken the once-bitten-twice-shy get-out route, but we are not like that. I always quote an old friend who once said to me 'life is not a dress rehearsal'. We don't get to the end and have the option to say, 'I liked that bit of my life, but next time round I'll change this or that'. There isn't a next-time-round for any of us. We all owe it to ourselves to make the very best of the one chance we get. To me there is nothing worse than wondering 'what if?', having never taken the opportunity to know for sure because you never even tried.

Yes, we could have taken the easy risk-free option and plodded on in our lives. But we are not plodders. We always need something to strive for, a dream to achieve.

Where would we be now if we had not strived for years on IVF? If we had not kept focused on the potential rewards of our efforts? I know the answer to that; we would have been a couple of 'childless plodders'. It's as though the successful conclusion to many years of struggle gave us the belief that together we can come through anything.

We lost a lot of money all those years ago when we had to close our shop. But I had realised a long-standing ambition when we opened it. I'm not sitting here today wondering what it would have been like owning my very own fashion business. Because I know. I experienced it. I can say I did it, not 'what if?'

Just because the outcome in the end was not the desired one does not take away the fact that we did it. You win some you lose some. IVF working for us was the one we won to prove my point.

Closing the shop did not signal the end of our world. Far from it. We were having a great life. Where would be the fun in getting everything you want the moment you desire it? Human beings need challenges, aims, objectives and a purpose for living. And suddenly here was something else to go for, another opportunity.

An opportunity to do what, exactly? Make a lot of money? Yes! Create a business? A new company? Yes! Improve our lifestyle? Certainly! Build that feeling of achievement and pride? Yes to all the above, but most crucially to Trudie and me now in our late 40s, it was the platform on which we could start to plan our retirement.

Our lives up until this point had been very much living for the now. Not in a frivolous fool-hardy way, but putting the distant future on hold and concentrating on attaining more immediate goals. Now we had reached the point where we could and should start looking further ahead. In fact we were well behind schedule in terms of conventional retirement planning, but the business plans looked sound and with the right sort of focus and effort there was every reason to believe we could start playing catch up very soon. And on that basis we embarked on yet another venture.

No Regrets

Lloyd:

It was decided that I would be the managing director of the new company. Not that titles matter to me one jot. I always say pay me the right money for a job I enjoy, and you can call me whatever you like. I'll also take on any tasks that are required to get the job done and in fact have no time for 'prima donnas' who think it's okay to hide behind a swanky title without applying the necessary work ethic. I'll get my hands dirty and work round the clock if that will pave the route to success. I'm focused and driven in everything I do.

I'll take calculated risks in business, but you try and think of any successful business person who has not taken a risk sometime.

Our optimism was not misguided as the new company turned over in excess of £1million in the first six months! During that time my feet never touched the ground as I covered over 30,000 miles of the country's roads attending meeting, conferences and seminars. From scratch I recruited and trained over 300 people to work to the required standard.

I'm not one for underestimating my own abilities. In fact I have been accused by some people of being arrogant. But the runaway early success of our business caught even me by surprise. It got to the stage where I was meeting myself coming back on a daily basis, and my family never saw me for weeks at a time. I used to joke that my son thought I was a burglar when he saw me coming in the front door on the rare occasions I was home!

Suffice to say I was putting heart, soul and everything I had into this opportunity, this retirement plan. The future looked so bright I needed shades.

Finally after all these years we were on track, not where we needed to be granted, but certainly heading in the right direction. Missing my family became the norm, but it was not going to be forever. When we did get time together it was quality time as I was earning more than I had ever earned before in my life and little trappings like the flashy motor were great perks. Nothing could go wrong.

I like to think I am a good judge of character. Correction, I am a good judge of character, a very good judge of character. I can sum up individuals within a very short time of meeting them and it's an uncanny ability that has served me well down the years.

I know when to get involved with individuals I come across on life's highway and I can suss out the sort of people who need to be given a wide berth. Only once in my whole life has this ability to spot 'the good, the bad or the ugly' ever let me down. And the consequences of that one little error were to prove potentially life-shattering.

The term 'con man', or to use the full title, 'confidence trickster' is often used to describe people who take advantage of others by pretending to be someone or something they are not in order to gain financially. As it alludes to in the name, the perpetrator behaves in a way that is calculated to give them credibility with their intended target. The victim starts to have 'confidence' in that person who in turn nurtures the growing trust to a point where they can do no wrong in the eyes of their intended target.

I used to read newspaper stories or see something in the news about someone who had been conned in some way and I would say, "What a stupid so-and-so, they deserve everything they got". Let's just say I no longer react like that when I hear of such incidents. Because I experienced at first hand how good a real confidence trickster can be.

I like to think I'm a very intelligent bloke, I'm street wise, I'm savvy, call it what you like, but I'm very sharp and as I said earlier I can spot a 'wrong 'un' coming in my direction. So how did I manage to get myself 'debagged' in broad daylight with my eyes wide open? Well, for a start I was way too busy making the business work to have doubts about the one person I thought was pulling 100% in the same direction as I was.

I was too busy to stop to cross all the t's and dot all the i's of the legal documents that would have protected me from my ultimate fate. There were far more pressing issues and we would get round to that sort of stuff at some stage, or so I thought. My business partner and 'great friend' of five years had other ideas. Looking back, he had other ideas that were formed long before he performed his coup de grace.

He knew all along that I could potentially make us millions, but he also knew from the start that he had no intention of sharing the spoils. To him I was just a means to a very carefully planned end.

It would be easy for me to say I lost everything. I did, if 'everything' was all the money I had pumped into the business, my six-figure salary and big car, our financial route to the future. I lost my credit rating practically overnight as my finances were on such a knife-edge to start with and my income just suddenly stopped.

It didn't take long before the creditors started getting their claws into us, but my son put the whole sorry affair into perspective one night when discussing it with his Mum. "He took away everything we want but left with us everything we need. We are all still here and we all love each other, that's all that matters".

Yes we do discuss things like that with our son, and yes he really did say that. That's the kind of lad he is. When Trudie told me I cried for the one and only time about the situation. I didn't cry for myself, I was hurting for my family. I was letting them down in my eyes, delivering yet another false dawn. But in their eyes I was as big a man as I had always been. They still loved me, I was still the best Dad and husband in the world and knowing how strongly they were behind me enabled me to keep my pride and dignity intact.

When you hit such a low point in your life and you start to think you are all alone in the world and there's practically no point in carrying on, you must stop and put things into perspective. My son was right. As young as he is, in fact probably because he is so young and not yet tainted by life's regular kicks in the nuts, he could see that all I had lost was material. Money and trinkets is not what life is all about. It's great to have enough to be comfortable but your whole life should not be about wealth and possessions.

We only need to look in the media to see how many celebrity relationships that are swimming in cash go pear-shaped in a very short space of time. Having pots of dosh does not necessarily make them happy relationships.

Pride plays a big part in how someone feels when they end up as I did. I took a massive blow to my ego and wanted to hide away from the world. Others go to more extremes and all too often we hear of tragic tales of someone who has taken their own life because they could not face up to the fact that they had lost a business or had come unstuck financially in some other way.

I never for a moment felt like that but I can understand how a person could be driven to those extremes if they did not have the love and support that I had.

Anyway I love myself and love my family far too much to ever consider taking my own life!

I still walk with my head held high as I have nothing to be ashamed of. I was badly wronged but everyday since I have dealt with it. I know I am a better person for the experience as I now have more time and compassion for others. It could be so easy to spend the rest of my years waiting and looking out for the next 'confidence trickster' to come along but we have moved on in our lives and the epitaph I had planned for my gravestone still reads the same. Two simple words.........

'NO REGRETS'

Bend Me
Over and
Cane Me!

Lloyd:

Over an hour I had been waiting to be called to the courtroom and now I was getting fed up. 'Just call me in, bend me over and cane me so I can then get on with the rest of my life', I was thinking, pretty much how I felt many years ago when I had to go and see the Head Master at school.

I was 14 years old and even though I went to a posh Grammar School I had somehow ended up mating around with the few bad apples that were in the same year as me. Like a set of complete morons we had decided it was a bit of a laugh to vandalise some property on the edge of the school grounds during our lunch break. The caretaker of the building we smashed up had chased us for miles before our youthful legs carried us to safety.

Or so I thought.

First lesson after lunch I got summoned out of class to go and see the Head Master.

I was shown into his office and he stood up from his desk, towering over me. He showed me a seat and very calmly asked me to sit down, which I immediately did. He followed suit and sat down in his huge, leather high-backed chair and towered over me even more.

He began to speak again, still calmness personified, and never once did he raise his voice. The conversation went thus…

"Thompson, I want you to give me the name of every boy that was with you when you decided to create mayhem and smash up the nature hut."

"Don't know what you're on about, Sir"...

"There were six of you seen hurling rocks through the windows, all wearing our school uniform, and I want their names!"

"No! Wasn't me Sir, like I said I don't know what you're on about".

"Thompson, you have been clearly identified as one of the culprits, causing destruction while wearing our school uniform, now tell the truth!"

"I am telling the truth! I wasn't there! I know nothing about it! No one saw me do anything!"

"Thompson! May I remind you, just in case it has slipped your attention, that you are the only black boy in this school?"...

Shit! I was rumbled, this was 1974 and yes, I was one of only two black kids in the whole school. My sister Yvonne, a year older, was the other. There was no getting out of it; no way could I claim mistaken identity on this one.

Suffice to say I sang like a canary from that point and may even have given names of lads who were not even there, but it still did not save me from getting the cane. Corporal punishment at schools was seen as acceptable in the 70s. I was facing expulsion, but my parents and previous good record saved me from that fate.

Maybe it was the wake-up call I needed as I managed to stay out of bother for the remainder of my school days.

But this wasn't school, this wasn't a Head Master I was about to face. I was going in to see a big scary judge, and just wanted it to be all over.

I had elected not to seek legal representation on the grounds that I did not want to throw good money after bad by paying someone to do something I felt fully capable of dealing with myself. I had read up on all the information that is readily available for people who find themselves in an IVA or bankruptcy situation and was confident in spite of my fear.

I did actually overhear a solicitor saying to another guy that the court used to deal with one or two bankruptcy cases a week and that this week already there had been 90. That, in just one of the many courts in this country. So I was not alone in my predicament, in fact it seemed almost fashionable to be a bankrupt.

I could see myself at dinner parties in the future... "What?! You mean to say you have never been a bankrupt? Oh, all the best people are doing it now darling... get with the programme, it's the latest must have 'social feather' to your cap!"...

"Calling Clinton Lloyd Thompson!"...

Talk about snapping out of a daydream.

This was it. Crunch time. I was going in to make it all official. I looked up to see who was addressing me by my full Sunday best moniker and saw the court official, a small, friendly-looking man standing in the doorway to one of the corridors that led off from the main waiting area. He was scanning the room to see who would answer. There was still time for me to high-tail it out of there, avoid the whole scary conclusion to my financial plight. But before my brain realised what my body was doing I found myself standing up and nodding towards the clerk in acknowledgement as his eyes landed on me.

Unlike at school many years ago I was owning up, first time round. I was the next bankrupt to be added to the list. He confirmed my details once more before I followed him the short distance to the allotted court-room.

As I entered the Court I sensed the 'officialdom' immediately. The atmosphere was very sombre; the judge was a tall, imposing character as he stood up behind a ridiculously huge desk to greet me.

We both sat down and he went straight into his summing up of my situation, as he understood it from my case notes.

I bet I was in there less than five minutes during which time he told me everything I already knew about where I stood. He just wanted acknowledgement from me that I fully appreciated what I was getting into and the long and short term consequences. But I had done my homework and fully grasped what to expect from this point.

He was duty- bound to point out that I could lose my home but I knew that not to be the case because of all the negative equity I was in. I started to explain this but he cut me short and told me he was not there in a specific advisory capacity, he was there to explain the law in general terms.

Before I knew it he declared me bankrupt and I was being shown out the door!

Wow! Was that it then? My whole financial life summed up and filed away under B for bankrupt in just five minutes. I was now just another statistic with my own bankruptcy reference number and everything. I had been allocated my prison uniform and I.D. number but I walked out of that court determined not to wear it with shame.

I felt strange walking from the Court building with my new-found status. Was it how I expected to feel? I wasn't sure, but I certainly felt different. I tried to sum up my thoughts and emotions. Was I scared? Was I angry? Was I bitter or resentful? No, I was experiencing none of these feelings as I made my way back to the car park.

So what was suppressing all the negative emotions that surely it would have been quite acceptable for me to be experiencing given what had just happened? Then it hit me, the climax of relief suddenly registered in my mind. My whole being started to relax as I realised the magnitude of weight that had been lifted from my very weary shoulders.

I was smiling and there was a definite spring in my step. I was not normal. How could I be feeling this way? Maybe I was experiencing 'post traumatic court disorder' or something? Should I not be fearing the worst for the future for myself and my family? But what was there to fear now? What more could be thrown at me?

That's why I was relieved, that's why I was smiling. I knew that without doubt I had come to the end of the financial rocky road.

Creditors could no longer call me any time night or day to harass me for money I did not have. Debt collectors would no longer come knocking at my door, scaring my wife and child and threatening me with dire consequences of non payment of monies owed. I would never again get any bills in the post.

We still had a roof over our heads and a car courtesy of the new company I was working for.

We were not destitute, living rough or going without life's essentials. We still had a future to look forward to, and that's why I was smiling.

I know that for many people the 'shame of bankruptcy' becomes a burden far too heavy to carry. It becomes a skeleton way back in the cupboard that must never be brought out and dusted off for public viewing. The temptation to 'hide your tracks' and carry on living as though nothing has happened must be overwhelming for some. But I never felt that way.

Surely to try and carry on living to the same life style as before could only lead to trouble again, as you would be living beyond your means.

Who are you trying to impress anyway? You have to take responsibility for the change in your circumstances and live within your capabilities. Observe and abide by the new parameters that have been set.

I know many of you will be thinking, 'but what will people think? What will your friends / family say?' 'Who gives a stuff!' is what I reply to that.

I gave up on the fight to win back my business, because I had no more money to line the pockets of the solicitors who are often the only winners at times like this.

I had long since waved off the transporter lorry as it drove off into the night with my dream car on top. It was the right thing to do as I could no longer afford to keep it.

We happily shop at Lidl every week, as opposed to Tesco, because we save money there. I only work with cash so that I can account for every penny I spend.

I notice the enquiring looks as I take my son on the school run, I can see them thinking, 'wonder what happened to the dream car?' But strangely no one ever asks out loud. Maybe it's a British thing, to wonder and to speculate but not dare to ask for fear of offending.

Ask me, I won't be offended. I'll be more than happy to tell you what's gone on in my life. My cupboard is bare, there are no skeletons.

People have to take me and mine for what we are. If what we are does not meet their approval then it's their problem not ours. We are a family that can look in the mirror and like what we see every morning we awake.

The Sum of

Our Choices

Lloyd:

It is said that we cannot chose what we are. Yet what are we but the sum of our choices in life.

Think about it and you start to realise how true this statement is. Apply it to yourself and consider what other choices you could have made in your life and where your choices have led you to at this point in time. What were the alternatives? Could you have made better choices, or are you like me living with no regrets?

As a black guy with a disability living in Britain my life could have been so very different if I had chosen it to be that way. I could be living a life full of regrets if I had let the wrong choices manifest. Let me explain…

I was born in this country to parents who came here in the 50's from Jamaica. They came here independently of each other, my mum in her teens and my dad in his early 20's, and I am still trying to get an answer to my question as to how two people could separately leave the tropical paradise that is Jamaica and manage to meet in Bolton, Greater Manchester? Anyhow, strange as it seems, that's what happened and they fell in love, married and had kids.

I'm the second of four, with an older sister and a younger brother and sister as siblings. When I was a toddler I had the misfortune to contract 'polio'. Not an illness you hear much about these days but it was rather too prevalent in the early 60's and I was one of the unlucky ones. Then again I was lucky too. Polio in most cases wastes the muscles in the legs, arms and sometimes attacks the spine, but in my case there was only a long lasting effect in my left arm, so I did not have to look forward to spending my whole life in a wheelchair. See, there's always a bright side if you look for it!

If you listen to my mother she will tell you that I started to make the right choices at a very early age. She will tell you that I quickly learned to start sticking up for myself, as opposed to being the 'poor little black boy with only one arm needing lots of sympathy'.

I actually started school in Jamaica when my parents took us out there for a couple of years, and by all accounts I had to get a new writing slate quite regularly to replace the one that I had broken on some foolhardy child who had tried to take liberties with me, thinking the one armed guy would be an easy target. I'm not suggesting for one minute that giving someone a good crack is the best way of settling a dispute, but when you are five years old you are not wise in the ways of arbitration, so my trusty slate board served me well in my infancy.

Why did my parents take us out to Jamaica? They were making good use of our very extended family. We lived with my Gran for a couple of years while my parents came back to Britain to continue working, and building a sound foundation on which to raise a family.

They were continuing where they had left off before having us kids. In short, they were both working very hard and doing whatever it takes to succeed. They were making sacrifices.

They had both arrived on these shores for the sole purpose of working. They were looking for opportunities that were not available in their homeland at that time. In fact, the British Government were very actively encouraging people to leave the West Indies to come and fill the thousands of job vacancies that existed as a result of a booming post-war Britain. The transport services in particular were desperate for workers because the indigenous population were either too few or not wanting the lower-paid manual jobs.

I don't think desperate is too strong a word to use, because my parents have told me about the recruitment campaigns that British companies ran in places like Kingston, making outlandish claims that the streets of Britain were 'paved with gold'!

When they arrived here they realised that the ad men had used artistic licence to the extreme. My mum still tells me now how 'grey' the country was. Grey sky, grey buildings and even grey people! She was just 15 years old and had been brought up on blue skies, sunshine and sea, and then wound up in Bolton. She says if it wasn't for the fact she'd spent her last penny getting here she would have jumped straight back on the next boat heading back out to the Caribbean. Turning tail and running away was not an option, so she had to get on with it. Find somewhere to live, find a job and start sending money 'back home', as being the eldest of 11 brothers and sisters she was expected to help provide for them from the riches she was going to gather in the land of 'golden pavements'.

More than 50 years on, although sadly not together anymore, both my parents are still here enjoying retirement, having contributed to this society by always working hard and paying their taxes and I'm now beginning to get to my point.

In the main I believe my parents made the right choices in life. They chose to come here in the first place, they chose not to turn tail and run when the going got tough. And I know it got very tough at times. They made the choices for us as kids, choices that meant we grew into the young adults we became and from there we were well schooled in the art of choosing. I don't want to speak for my brother and sisters, but I like to think my own resilience, optimism for life and bounce-back-ability must be largely down to my parents. And be it consciously or sub-consciously, I have developed a knack of making the right choices.

Living Off a
Perceived
Disability...

Lloyd:

Yes, I have a disability, but don't ever dare call me 'disabled' because I am able enough to do anything I set my mind to. I have never registered myself as disabled or stated on any job application that I am disabled. I have never been out of work because I choose not to be and consequently never claimed a penny from the state. I drive a car as long as it's automatic and I have always been active in sport, from football to swimming. A mate once asked me how come I don't go round in circles when I swim. Was I offended? No, it's one of the funniest things I've ever heard!

Other people have asked how come I'm not registered disabled because I could claim disability allowance. Now I'm really getting to the point I want to make. Why the hell would I want to sit around on my arse all day living off the back of a 'perceived disability', while other hard-working tax payers provide for me? As I keep saying, it's about making choices, and I chose to work for a living and contribute to society, like my parents always did. Too many people these days look for the easy option of sponging off the state, and I know there are people out there who would love to have my 'disability' because of how much it could boost their claim from the Social! I'm not exaggerating; I know professional scroungers who have boasted of their knowledge on how 'the system' works, giving me tips on how best I could take advantage of it to get 'free money'. This is a system that champions hair-brained schemes such as making the internet available for all. In theory a great ideal to hold, in practice if you are on benefits you can claim your free laptop with internet connection set up for you but, if you are stupid enough to be working and earning just enough to survive then it's tough luck if you can't afford to be hooked up to the wonderful 'worldwide web'. Then again I suppose we can all send our kids to play at the houses of the kids whose parents are unemployed so that they can use their computers and watch their giant plasma TV's, presuming they're not away on one of their many holidays!

It sounds like I'm joking but the sad thing is that I'm being deadly serious. These people have spent their lives making the wrong choices and are conditioned to think the way they do. The idea of working for a living is not even a consideration; they actually believe they are owed a living.

If back in the 1970's you'd have told my parents that their 'black disabled son' would grow up to be a Conservative voter they would have felt that they had made some grave errors in the way they raised me, mostly because the Tories were seen as the party that did not welcome immigrants into Britain due to the likes of Enoch Powell. West Indians always voted Labour as a direct result of that. So why am I bucking the trend and voting Tory? It's because the Labour Government we have had for the past 13 years is way too keen on aiding and abetting the 'scrounging, layabout society'.

I'm not talking about genuine cases here. Some people through no fault of their own cannot work and deserve every bit of help and support we can give them from the system. I'm talking about those who choose not to work, those who make a lifestyle choice to be a scrounger and layabout. Those who if they woke up one morning black and disabled would think they had won the lottery. Even better if they had kids as well, because the 'State' won't see kids going hungry or homeless, so the more kids you have the more free money you can get your hands on.

What does any of this have to do with IVF or bankruptcy you may wonder? Well, I'm just making the point that there are two extreme ways in which children are viewed here. Some people see kids as a means to a financial end, as a passport to gaining a Council house and regular work-free income. They have plenty of time on their hands because they choose not to work. Yet none of that time or money that they claim is devoted to their kids, who are left to bring themselves up, roaming our streets and getting into trouble while the layabout parents sit at home watching Jeremy Kyle and smoking and drinking the fags and booze paid for from my taxes. Then as the kids grow up, the whole depressing cycle starts all over again because these kids have not been brought up to make the right choices.

While on the other hand you have people like Trudie and me who actually went into debt in an effort to start a family, where all the years of trying and disappointment has given us a real appreciation of our child and family values and motivates us to be the best parents we can be.

We have morals and standards that hopefully will be instilled in Jayjay and enable him to make the right choices in his life.

I must have been a little naïve before becoming a parent because it's only since Jayjay became old enough to start playing out with other kids and going to their houses that I slowly started to become really aware of the 'layabout society'. Up until then it was not something I even thought about. I knew there were people out there who chose not to work when really they could, but I thought they were a very small silent minority. But there are loads of them and they are far from silent.

My son has friends whose parents do not work because of various illnesses and disabilities, but strangely these ailments don't stop them from getting down to the pub most nights or indeed flying off on the frequent holidays some of them seem to be comfortably able to afford from my taxes. I work damned hard for a living yet I can't remember the last time I went away on holiday. Maybe I'm the stupid one here, it could be argued, but I have pride, morals and too much self respect to take my family down that route.

So why do the scroungers do it? Answer... because they can. Because our benefits system plays straight into their hands, making it far too easy for them to claim, no questions asked, no real accountability on their part is required and it could be so very different.

What if in order to claim, these people had to face the tax-payers whose money they were pissing up the wall, as opposed to just sitting around waiting for the money to be paid into their bank accounts by faceless benefits agents? We could cut out the middle men, the civil servants, of which there are far too many anyway, and give our taxes direct to our allocated 'dole buddy'.

Yes, the first big saving the country would make under my 'dole buddy' scheme would be by cutting back on the armies of DSS employees apparently needed to make sure the slackers get their dough every week.

Just tell me who my allocated scrounger is and each month that I get paid (yes, they would have to wait a month like most other people); I will meet them at a pre-arranged place to give them their money. At that meeting I will agree with them the jobs they need to do for me in order to keep qualifying for my hand-out.

They could do my garden every couple of weeks, they could get my shopping and clean my windows or paint my house or carry out any of the tasks that I don't have time to do because I'm too busy working for 'our' money.

I would insist that my 'dole buddy' provides receipts to account for how my 'taxes' are being spent and while I would expect to see evidence of spending on food, fuel and other essentials to living, there is no way they would be allowed to spend my money on fags or booze. In other words, abuse the system and your money stops. It's about making these people have a sense of responsibility to our society.

You didn't think I was just going to give them my 'hard-earned' without some sort of payback? How long do you think it would be before the penny dropped and the humiliation got too much and our 'dole buddies' decided they may as well get a job?. Even if they didn't, at least we would be getting something in return for keeping them.

In reality a scheme such as 'dole buddies' would never get off the ground regardless of how much sense it makes. First of all the senior civil servants would never sanction something that would see their numbers diminish, and in this world of 'political correctness' I know my views will be seen by many as at the very least harsh, or by some as victimisation of the 'needy'. However, let's get back to the issue of bringing children into the world and the many different reasons and motivations we have for being parents.

For many starting a family is simply doing what comes naturally. Boy meets girl, they fall in love, get engaged, then married, buy a house and a Ford Mondeo then fill the house with 2.5 children and a golden retriever before going on to live happily ever after working 9-5 in order to maintain the status quo.

Then there are the people like us who plan to do what comes naturally only to find that getting pregnant is not quite as easy as falling off a log. Although strangely, I have never known or heard of anyone who would qualify as a 'dole buddy' struggling with infertility. 'Shelling them like peas' is usually the description connected with the scroungers.

Whatever the reason for wanting kids no one can deny that in order for the world to keep turning the human race must continue to procreate. Generation has to follow generation. As we age and retire then eventually die we need newer and younger generations to replace us and continue working and running the world. Countries like ours need great kids to become the teachers, scientists and politicians of the future. We should be doing our utmost to make sure that once we bring children into the world we equip them not just to survive but to contribute to society.

I have already said that there are too many people who have kids for all the wrong reasons, and as a result have no interest whatsoever in bringing up these kids with the right moral fibre to play a decent part in our social infrastructure. And I truly believe that.

I also believe just as strongly that most couples with the determination to combat infertility and subject themselves to all the traumas of the whole process are looking to produce offspring for all the right reasons. You don't go through all that trouble and expense in order to get yourself further up the waiting list for a Council flat.

So here's the big dilemma - although it should be such an easy choice - does the Government continue to be hoodwinked into supporting people who have children for all the wrong reasons, or do the politicians open their eyes, realise what's going on and start giving more to IVF funding and helping people who want kids for all the right reasons? Do we help the people who are looking to produce and nurture worthy offspring, or continue to give handouts to the ones who are looking to breed children purely for the immediate benefits of housing and handouts without a thought to that child's future? These are the poor soles that the NSPCC are requesting just £2 a month to save!

We then moan and groan about 'kids today' when we witness the mayhem they can cause in our towns and cities on a Friday night, but is it any wonder when you stop to consider the start in life that many of them have had?

Why should the process of applying for welfare payments be easier than the 'Spanish Inquisition' type ordeal we and many others have to go through to justify our wish to have children? Like I say, I have never applied for benefits so I can't claim to have first hand knowledge, but from speaking to people who have, I know there's not too much demand placed on applicants to prove they are worthy recipients of our hard-earned yet never seen taxes going straight into the system.

Before we could be accepted on to the NHS funded IVF programme we had to fill out countless numbers of forms and then be interviewed by doctors, specialists and even councillors to make sure we were of sound mind and worthy of benefiting from the tiny pool of money that is allocated to IVF from the system.

Then, unlike claiming from the DSS you are limited on how much funding you can have. Three attempts then that's your lot. If you have not been fortunate enough to conceive before the money runs out its tough luck, because from that point you're on your own. Why is that sort of ultimatum not given to individuals claiming benefits? Why can we not say, 'you can claim for x number of months or claim x amount of pounds, and then if you are not in work by then you are on your own'?

What rankles with me is the fact that Trudie and I have paid far more into the system than we were ever given on IVF before funding was stopped, while too many people who claim benefits have paid in very little, if anything at all, and it seems that they can go on claiming forever and a day without anyone challenging 'their right' to do so.

There is an argument that says everyone living in this country in the 21st century has a right to expect a decent standard of living i.e. above the breadline as a very minimum, and I don't argue against that point for a second. What I will argue is my belief that every couple has the right to be parents; every woman should be able to experience pregnancy and child birth if that's what she wants. Having children is a basic and natural instinct that should not be denied anyone who is fit and proper and equipped to carry out the most important job any of us ever undertakes. And the IVF procedure ensures that all these checks are in place while in a very perverse and unjust way our benefits system encourages people who would never get through IVF, because they would fall at the first hurdle to have as many kids as they can, and bring them up on tax-payers' money that could, and should, be routed to a much worthier cause!

After the Bomb

Trudie:

After we lost our business we all felt the huge shock and devastation but as always we tried to be brave and cheerful to give encouragement and support to one another. We always back each other 100%, 100% of the time and this somehow has always come naturally to us. I was mortified that something this horrific could have happened to someone as hardworking and diligent as Lloyd. His dream was ripped from him in the blink of an eye.

We were so busy working towards the end goal I suppose we were 'lambs to the slaughter'! Lloyd's brilliant idea, my contacts, the drive we both possessed, coupled to the ability to pull the whole thing together; we truly didn't see it coming. We threw ourselves whole heartedly into this project because we believed that this was the 'biggy'. This was how we were to secure the rest of our lives. This was how we were going to pay off our mortgage and when the company was up and running it was the plan to sell it, then we'd wander off into the sunset – Total Bliss! Well that was the plan and as far as we were concerned we were all working our wee tushes off in order to attain the same goal.

So when Hiroshima hit, it hit us at a million miles an hour and there was no protection whatsoever. There was nowhere to run and there was certainly nowhere to hide we just had to roll with the blows. We were stripped of everything. All of a sudden Lloyd wasn't bringing home the huge salary we were used to. My main concern was how was this going to affect my beautiful son. We were pretty much, how you'd say, head first in the poop!

Originally Lloyd had been given the title of managing director which made little impression on him, but he'd been given it so he wore it, and very well at that. I was very proud of him. He's never been a man for titles he's always been driven by money and securing our future always looking out for us. Always wanting to protect us and protect the future. Mind you he does have his weaknesses – Cars! Our motivation had only ever been to make as much money as possible so that we could pay off our mortgage, and secure maybe some kind of pension. Pretty much what everyone wants I'd imagine.

In the past we'd re-mortgage our property in order to fund the IVF. We also re-mortgaged to open up a menswear boutique in the late 80's, which I hasten to add was a phenomenal shop. We sold exquisite hand-picked designer menswear imported from Europe. The shop was stupendous and it took our minds off our fertility problems at that time. We threw ourselves into it and it became our baby for all intents and purposes. It took up all our time, I ran the shop under Lloyd's guidance and he carried on working for one of the multinationals. Though he was only going to stay in his position until Lapel Clothing Co had secured its second year of trading.

In the year that we were fortunate enough to have the shop we had a ball. We made lots and lots of interesting acquaintances; we could fill a book with the tales of running and owning a shop like ours. We laughed, we cried and we managed to pay all our bills but unfortunately due to the economic climate at that time we needed to close it down. We were lucky because there were numerous takers wanting a piece of Lapel so it didn't take long to off load it's heavy burden.

The end was a very sad time in our lives; I remember shutting the shop on the last night. We locked the door, we stood back and looked up at it and as we walked the mile or so home Lloyd, ever the philosopher, was still smiling and very cheery. He told me that he was happy that we'd given the shop a 'go' as he'd dreamt of owning his own boutique for years, he obviously was disappointed that all our hard-work hadn't managed to make it the roaring success we'd both hoped for but he was going down the route of 'better to have loved and lost than never to have loved at all' and for his part he was happy that he'd given it a go. So he pulled me out of my depression with his bright cheerfulness and I always remember him saying 'what doesn't kill you girl, makes you stronger'! He could now tick it off his 'life's list' of projects and he could crack on with the next challenge. I adored his 'glass half-full' attitude, I'd never met anyone with such enthusiasm and his optimism knew no bounds.

We both took on two jobs in order to regroup and repay the deficit we now owed. Unfortunately dreams do come with a price tag! We got our heads down and we ate lots of beans on toast and jam sandwiches, we found out that we were pretty good at tightening our belts.

A year after closing the shop we'd cleared our debts so I could breathe again, I hate owing money.

Lloyd was by now careering all around the country in his efforts to build the new company and he was over in Ireland too. He was holding seminars' in order to attract the sales staff for the new business. This proved to be another of his fortes and he shone like the superstar he is. I knew he was tired but all the success he was having was driving him on. I found in this period that we were both so busy; one week would just merge into another. Every night we'd get our 'good night' call from Daddy and he would listen in to the bedtime story, it was quite lovely actually, we were all very good at making the best of any situation. It was a walk in the park!

I took on the role of single parent. I was working 9.30hrs to 14.30hrs daily so I could accommodate each side of the school run but on the occasions I couldn't make it my lovely parents would step into the breach. They were very good at that. They never complained and they always made you feel that you were doing them a favour. I remember Lloyd once commenting that if they were to teach their parenting skills to the world, it really would be a wonderful place, never have two people been so selfless.

Though our lives were frantic we were like a couple of teenagers. We didn't care how much effort it took we were on one of the best journeys, some of the time it was a little bumpy, a little hare-em-scare-em, some of the time it ran like clockwork. It was only a matter of time before we'd be able to sit back, put our feet up and enjoy! Life was sweet! Or so we thought...

I remember the Sunday morning that we took the phone call that would destroy our dreams but funnily enough not our lives. Lloyd went to a 'thrown together last minute' meeting and it was there that he was to be dealt his/our fate. He was mortified to find he had no claim on his Company; he was to lose it all! Lloyd thought it must have been some kind of mistake, one that could be easily rectified. But there was no mistake! Piece by piece the whole sordid nightmare began to unfold. We had lost everything, well, almost. Lloyd was his usual tower of strength even on the day that the phones were cut off and his precious car was taken back. I remember him standing there saluting it off and my heart ached so much for him.

Lloyd bounced back into the house and began to surf the net and make calls to old acquaintances trying desperately to find a job to bridge our financial gap. The following morning he walked to the train station and I can remember his quip, "public transport is befitting of my new status – that of a bankrupt"!

As we were stripped of our belongings I prayed and prayed with all my might that we wouldn't lose our precious home and I somehow knew, deep down, that we wouldn't. Even in my darkest hour I held strong to the belief that we would survive this ordeal just as we'd survived the ordeals of the past.

We kept each other strong, and I include our beautiful son in that statement, he was like a shining beacon, he is so sensible, kind and caring. He approached me one day, "Mum can I ask you a question?" I turned to him, "Absolutely sweetheart what's up?" I knelt down so that our eyes were at a similar level and he began, "Mum, did you forgive the man who did this to Dad?" Wow, what a question, how do you answer that, then the words just came, "Of course I did honey and I went one better than that, I forgave myself for hating him because hate is such a negative emotion and the only person hate destroys is the person bothering to hate." I knew Lloyd would have been proud of that reply and for the life of me I had no idea where it came from but I was so glad it made such sense. We became quiet for a minute or two whilst Jayjay digested my answer, when I added "Right back at ya little un, did you forgive?" His reply completely floored me. "Yes Mum, but it took a long time…", (I hasten to add at this stage, that it had only been nine months since losing everything!) He continued, "… I sat on my bed one night and I asked myself what exactly did we lose? I came up with the fact that we only lost everything we WANTED but we were left with everything we needed – we are all still here!"

What a powerful statement from anyone let alone a nine year old boy and I know adults that wouldn't be as mature in a situation such as ours. How lucky was I? And yes, I had everything I needed right here. In fact it was fun bringing a quilt downstairs to keep us all warm of a winters evening, even friends would join in and snuggle under the quilt whilst watching TV, it became quite chic.

One of the saddest moments for me came one day just as Jayjay and I were about to leave for work and school, Lloyd appeared at the top of the stairs in his pj's and as he descended the staircase he started, "Before you both leave I owe you an apology." What was he talking about? "I've let you both down. I didn't keep you safe and that's the one thing I'm supposed to do, I'm a failure…." These words from my Lloyd, the most positive man in the world! Before he could add anymore I quickly stopped him in his tracks, "You don't owe anyone an apology, least of all us. We love you, we're proud of you and I for one know that you had to lose your company in order to attain your next goal which will be bigger and better. I'm excited about our future. Remember, we're the Thompson's and we're indicative of the musketeers, we stick together come rain or shine". By now he was on the bottom stair, the sun was shining through the window and across his face, for the very first time in his life he looked aged, he looked broken and I wondered how on earth I was going to hold us altogether. I didn't know how but I prayed I'd be shown a way.

We held onto each other, all three of us recharging our batteries, but we weren't weak and I for one had great faith that from your darkest hour you would be given, or should I say you would be shown, your greatest gift just as George Bailey had in It's A Wonderful Life!

There were many sad and poignant moments, like the time I arrived home to find a letter from Jayjay's bank explaining that all the money in his savings account had been impounded due to the fact that Lloyd's name was on his passbook. My heart just stopped. How could I resolve this? My mind galloped around looking for the answer. They had taken his £200.00 which he'd been diligently saving for computer equipment. All his Christmas money and his birthday money. My poor sweet boy. My little trouper who no longer even bothered asking for anything as he was well aware of our dire situation. My lovely son was now being persecuted because of his father's great misfortune. How totally unfair. I managed to hold myself together and started to prepare our evening meal. Jayjay had gone out to play football with friends and do what little boys do best, have fun. As I began to cook I reached for the phone and rang Lloyd. He was mortified, "Leave it with me, I'll speak to the Official Receiver in the morning, I promise I'll get his money back!"

I turned the radio on hoping that some music would ease my distress. Van Morrison's 'Have I told you lately that I love you', crooned out and totally took my breath away. Whenever Jayjay heard this tune he would always ask me to dance with him, he called it 'our song'. Tears poured down my cheeks as I returned to the kitchen. I was really struggling. I wasn't sobbing but I was close. All of a sudden a hand touched my shoulder, "They're playing our song mum. Could I have this dance?" Jayjay had returned and I hadn't even heard him. How could I turn round? "Absolutely!" was all I managed in the brightest voice I could muster. I was careful not to let him see my face and I held him so close. He sang every word as he always did. I was determined to retrieve his money. He would never know. I was not prepared to let him down – there just had to be a way.

Until this very day Jayjay never knew this part of our story and, yes, Lloyd managed to retrieve his money and I for one, am eternally grateful to our Official Receiver for all his help and guidance in moments like this, and believe me moments like that came along fast and furious there are far to many to list but suffice to say he always knew what to do and gave me lots of confidence in our ability to solve these little hiccups.

NHS &

Obesity

Lloyd:

Even when the NHS does manage to get it's hands on some money because thankfully not all of it goes to the 'dole scroungers', there are no guarantees that this money will be wisely spent. I know I could easily be accused of being biased in favour of all things IVF but even without our experiences of infertility I'm sure I would still be getting on my next 'Hobby Horse' of complaint. What the hell is he finding to beef about now you may be thinking? I'll tell you. The latest scourge of our great nation - obesity, and the ever increasing number of people who think its okay to stuff pies, chips, cake, chocolate and all manner of junk food into their mouths as if food was going to run out tomorrow! Not only that, obese people who would never consider exercise to counter the balance of the thousands of calories that they pile in everyday. These are the ones who take full advantage of the fact that most pizza-parlour's and curry-houses will now deliver free of charge as long as you are spending enough money on your order. "Walk to the chippy and collect your feast?" Or am I just being too ridiculous to even suggest that!

Do you know that the NHS spent £50m in 2009 treating obesity? 50 million big ones were spent pandering to the crazy notion that it's never the fault of the individual. It's the food manufacturers, supermarkets and fast food establishments who are to blame if some arguments were to be believed and all overweight people deserve help to shed the results of their gross over-indulgence across the years.

I know I run the risk of offending overweight people everywhere but maybe you need to be offended so that you can wake up to the fact that being overweight in 99% of cases is down to one simple equation and that is if you put into your body more than you burn up then you are going to put on weight. Fact! Plain and simple fact. Don't talk to me about thyroids and hereditary conditions. Chances are the only thing you have inherited is your parent's capacity for tucking away the wrong types of foods in great quantity because fat parents do tend to breed fat kids and that's not fair on the kids who are young and impressionable and look up to their parents for guidance and follow their lead. If they are going to bring their kids up on fast-foods and stodgy rubbish while allowing them to sit on their 'Play Stations' all day long because they can't be bothered to take them swimming or down the park then they are literally contributing to the next generation of obese adults.

This all goes back to the topic of 'choices' I mention earlier in this book. They are choosing to have kids then not do right by them. They are building up problems that are potentially life threatening for their kid's future and what sort of parenting is that?

I must sound like I hate overweight people but truth is I don't hate anyone in this world, even those who have greatly wronged me and my family. This particular topic gets under my skin because it's another one of those that I can route back to the lack of funding in IVF. £50M could pay for 7,000 IVF treatments per year and while many of those treatments would ultimately come to nothing as we so painfully and personally know, there would still be thousands more babies being born to parents who want them for the right reasons and who would not spend their time fattening them up like Christmas turkeys.

So how is the NHS spending our taxes to fight obesity? They are spending £10k to £12k per time fitting 'gastric bands' in order to shrink the stomachs and therefore eating capacity of clinically obese patients. Now if I'm not mistaken, the need to shrink a person's stomach in order to reduce the amount of food they can eat would suggest that person tends to shovel in too much food, so nothing whatsoever to do with thyroids or hereditary conditions, it's to combat pure greed and self-indulgence and nothing else.

Other monies are also being spent on giving these people free liposuction. What a great message that sends out. It's okay to stuff yourself to the point of death then pop down to your local GP with your sob story of how 'life is so unfair because I only eat a lettuce leaf and a stick of celery each day and because my thyroid is under active I keep gaining weight', then he'll arrange to get your excess fat sucked out courtesy again of our taxes!

How, I often wonder, does anyone get to the point of being 25, 30 or 40 stone in weight before they realise things are critical and something needs to be done? Surely at some point previously they have known they need to do something about their obesity? You would think so but more often than not it takes some major embarrassing incident to trigger a reaction. Something like getting stuck in a turnstile at a football stadium or having to book two seats on an aeroplane because they cant fit into one. Although according to a Joan Rivers joke they are pacified by the fact that booking two seats means they get two meals on the plane. And there you have another 'side effect' of obesity. Yes obese people are an easy target for jokers' worldwide. Is that what any of us wants and more particularly is that what any of us want for our children? To always be the butt of the joke, being singled out as different simply because of their weight? We all know how cruel kids can be to each other so why put your offspring at an early disadvantage in life when you can choose not to?

Now I'm sure I'm not the only one to have heard stories in the news of people being refused routine operations because they have been overweight and the surgeons have been concerned that the patient may suffer heart failure on the operating table. It's also true to say that women who are overweight are not allowed to start an IVF programme. So how come these concerns are put to one side when carrying out major surgery such as a gastric bye pass? Surely the safer option would be for these people to get some self discipline and control in their lives and eat in moderation and take a stroll now and again?

Yes make them show willing. Make them demonstrate by their actions that spending our taxes on them won't be a waste of time, resources and money. For example if someone needs to lose 20st.

they should have to lose the first 3 or 4st. themselves by way of sensible eating and exercise. If they can achieve their target then fair enough they get the operation. If they can't be disciplined enough to take those first few steps alone then why should we waste time and money giving them the lazy way out? Just by applying some common sense like this you would see the number of people qualifying for gastric bands or lipo decrease dramatically I would bet!

The recent story that really brings my point home is of the woman weighing over 40st who was in hospital having treatment for her obesity. The tax payers, you and I, had already forked out thousands to help this woman and in the end she died because she was putting pressure on her family to sneak food into the hospital for her and they, being equally as weak, obliged with pizzas and fish 'n' chips until she literally ate herself to death.

Even more recently it has been suggested that cash incentives should be offered to obese people to encourage them to lose weight and to smokers to entice them into giving up! Pass me the fried chicken and a pack of 20, I'm getting on this latest gravy train!

I'm not claiming to be the man with all the answers because it's a tough job making our benefits and healthcare systems work. I do however believe that 'common sense' is greatly lacking when the big wigs making the decisions on 'who gets what' sit round the table.

Surely they are not so naïve as to think all the people getting the pounds are worthy candidates. There is enough money in the pot if only it went to the right places and for the right reasons and giving money to those who have abused their own bodies by over eating at the expense of other more worthy causes is not right.

An even more recent incident of blatant abuse of the system caught my attention this week. A guy has asked his GP to refer him on to have a gastric band fitted to help him lose weight. However it turns out that his 'body mass index' is below the level required for the procedure to be given the OK. Now my first thought would be 'oh maybe I'm not as overweight as I thought, I'll try and get the weight off myself'... even if ultimately I tried and failed I would look to give it a go but that's not the thought pattern of the hero in this story. No! He's going in completely the opposite direction. He has stated his intention to 'beef up'. Yes that's right, he intends to feast on as much fatty food as he can until he reaches the weight required to qualify for having a gastric band fitted! How do the minds of these people work? How is he being allowed to get away with it? He should be told that if that's the way he wants to treat his body then he is disqualified from having the treatment, end of story.

I don't suppose the Government would want to adopt another policy of mine to go with 'Dole Buddies'? it's quite a simple one really... just pass a law that forces any fast food establishment to do away with their delivery service and in addition they also have to have narrow doorways to their shops. That's right a pre-determined maximum width of entrances for everyone selling 'Fat Food'! This would mean that first of all everyone would have to go and collect their own food but if on arrival at the shop they could not fit through the doorway then they could not go in and buy the grub. I've already spotted the flaw in this scheme however in that most of them would just hang around outside waiting for a skinny person to go in and get their food for them. Well it was just a thought. A thought better than the idea of paying them not to eat so much at least!

The Gift of Choice

Choice n. choosing; opportunity or power of choosing; thing or person chosen; possibilities from which to choose. –adj. of superior quality.

The above is the 'Collins English Dictionary' definition of one of the most under-rated things we all have available to us in our lives. We all have choices to make practically by the day, hour, minute and second. We are called upon to make hundreds of decisions or choices as I prefer to call them everyday. Now thankfully the majority of choices we have to make are automatic ones in response to any manner of minor incidents that can crop up on life's highway and we make our decisions and deal with the situation without even thinking about it.

However, life as we know is not all plain sailing. Life throws up far more than the little day-to-day incidents that can be dealt with while our minds are on automatic pilot.

Every now and then we are required to switch off the auto pilot and take the controls because we are experiencing some turbulence or need to plot another route on our life journey.

Most people would read this as taking control because there is a problem or some adversity to deal with. This is where most people would be wrong.

Instead of seeing a problem or an adversity, see it as an opportunity. See it as a chance to do whatever you want from that point on. Chose what it is you want to do or achieve. Don't think to yourself, 'Oh I have this major problem to deal with and it's beyond me'.

Instead think, "I have in front of me a fantastic opportunity to..." then fill in the blanks!

Whatever the perceived problem, you have an opportunity to make choices. You have the opportunity to make a difference.

I'm just an ordinary person. Trudie and Jayjay are ordinary people too but we have achieved some extra ordinary things in our lives through the power of self-belief and believing in each other. We always trust in our ability to make the right choices in order to explore the opportunities that come our way.

Infertility and IVF was not a 'problem' it was an opportunity for Trudie and me to really get to know each other as a couple over those 12 years. It was a time in which we grew to really appreciate what it would mean to have a baby and raise a child worthy of his place on this earth. We had time to mature and experience life and as a result we will always be able to guide our son and offer advice to him based on our life experiences. We know without a shadow of doubt that he will grow up to be a credit to us and more importantly a credit to himself and he will make a difference to the world, well equipped to make good choices. After all he's already demonstrated his fighting spirit before he was even born because when Trudie was in labour with him and the umbilical cord was wrapped around his neck it really was a case of 'life or death' yet he overcame that hurdle to begin his life.

The IVF years were also an opportunity for Trudie to really discover herself. I don't think she had any idea what a strong, determined and focused person she was when we set out on that journey. Yet time and again she amazed me and herself by bouncing back to try again after every failure. She never chose to give up!

Trudie:

Whilst writing this, my father's partner gave me a book called 'The Secret' by Rhonda Byrne, it is a book I believe everyone should read and inwardly digest. Its message is so powerful and as I read through the words that Lloyd and I have written I realise how true Rhonda's book is. She says that the Law of Attraction is working all the time whether you are conscious of it or not. This is based on the principal that 'Like begets like', positive behaviour brings about more positive behaviour etc. etc. I am amazed at how many positive things the Law of Attraction as brought into my life, first there was Lloyd, then there was my beautiful Jayjay, there was the wonderful experience of Better Homes... and the list goes on. So I would like to thank you for that book I only wish I'd had it before I started on my IVF years.

St Mary's Hospital

Trudie and Lloyd Thompson are donating a percentage of the royalties from book sales to the St Mary's Hospital "Test tube baby IVF" charitable endownment fund, number 629364.

This fund was established to support and facilitate the scientific and clinical development of the Reproductive Medicine Department at St. Mary's Hospital Manchester.

It is a not-for-profit endowment that is administered by the Central Manchester University Hospitals NHS Foundation Trust.

The endowment supports scientific enquiry into novel and innovative methods of improving the effectiveness and safety of assisted conception and has been instrumental in the Department achieving its successful robust research profile.

It also provides support for Departmental Staff to acquire knowledge and skills for the improvement and advancement of assisted conception services. The field of assisted conception is a rapidly evolving one with regular updates in techniques and processes that require visits to other centres, conferences and meetings. This endowment partly supports St Mary's staff in these important activities.

The endowment furthermore supports the introduction of new equipment and ways of working into the Department and over the years these have led to huge gains in the clinical service and ultimately in improved treatment outcomes for the direct benefit of patients.

Lightning Source UK Ltd.
Milton Keynes UK
UKOW050627031211

183041UK00001B/5/P